DRUGS IN AMERICAN LIFE

Edited by Morrow and Suzanne Wilson

THE REFERENCE SHELF
Volume 47   Number 1

THE H. W. WILSON COMPANY   •   New York   •   1975

THE REFERENCE SHELF

The books in this series contain reprints of articles, excerpts from books, and addresses on current issues and social trends in the United States and other countries. There are six separately bound numbers in each volume, all of which are generally published in the same calendar year. One number is a collection of recent speeches; each of the others is devoted to a single subject and gives background information and discussion from various points of view, concluding with a comprehensive bibliography. Books in the series may be purchased individually or on subscription.

Library of Congress Cataloging in Publication Data

Wilson, Morrow, comp.
  Drugs in American life.

  (The Reference shelf ; v. 47, no. 1)
  Bibliography: p.
  1. Drug abuse--United States--Addresses, essays,
lectures. 2. Drug abuse--Social aspects--United States
--Addresses, essays, lectures. 3. Drugs--Laws and
legislation--United States--Addresses, essays, lectures.
I. Wilson, Suzanne, joint comp. II. Title.
III. Series. [DNLM: 1. Drug abuse--Collected works.
2. Drug and narcotic control--United States--Collected
works. WM270 W751d]
HV5825.W534   362.2'93'0973   75-4607
ISBN 0-8242-0569-3

PREFACE

The recent "drug scene" in the United States has been the subject of great discussion and controversy since it first became a matter of general concern in the middle 1960s. This volume is intended, primarily, for college and high school students, and the emphasis here is on youthful involvement with and approach to drugs. However, the use of drugs in one form or another, with or without general approval, has been a part of most societies since the beginning of recorded history. It may be helpful, therefore, to attempt to put the present drug situation in this country into historical perspective and to include discussion of other kinds of drug users besides youthful Americans.

The first section consists of three selections which, together, comprise an overview. Each article examines the drug phenomenon from a different point of view.

The second section deals with the legal aspects of drug use, addiction, possession, and sale in the United States in this century, insofar as it is possible to isolate legal aspects from others. Although the specific laws vary in different states, the general approach has been the same, as have been the pitfalls and problems.

The third and central section is difficult to summarize briefly. It includes discussions of many of the consciousness-altering substances, legal and illegal, that are common in American life, from a social or medical point of view. Also dealt with are the serious addictive drugs and the problems arising from their abuse. That overworked, and often misunderstood, term *abuse* can be defined as the use of any substance in such a way, and to such an extent, as to jeopardize the user's health, working life, or general welfare. Of course, drug abuse is often symptomatic of other serious socioeconomic difficulties or problems of adolescence. But

3

drug addiction does its own damage, and it becomes hard to tell which is cause and which is effect.

Most writing on the subject of drugs is done by professionals in one field or another—law, social work, medicine, psychology; with the exception of Dr. Andrew Weil, whose medical training and personal drug experimentation are combined in his work, most experts either do not have, or do not assert, direct personal involvement with drugs. It seems appropriate, therefore, to include, as the fourth section of this book, several personal accounts of subjective physical, mental, and emotional reactions to various drugs. The narrators—several acclaimed in their own professions— present not the wide-ranging views of drug experts but perceptive, moving records of individual experience.

The fifth and final section consists of a number of solutions to the drug problem. All the approaches have in common an optimistic attitude and an appeal for understanding of the situation and of its victims—the better to deal intelligently and effectively with it.

The editors wish to thank the publishers and authors who have granted permission to reprint selections in this compilation.

MORROW AND SUZANNE WILSON

January 1975

CONTENTS

V. Possible Solutions

I. OVERVIEW

EDITORS' INTRODUCTION

The three articles in this section offer three widely differing approaches to the present drug situation in the United States. It should be noted, too, that even terminology may be a source of confusion. Medically, narcotic drugs are those (such as opiates and barbiturates) that dull the senses and induce sleep or stupor; legally, however, the term *narcotic* has been applied to any drug (for example, the stimulant cocaine) thought to produce addiction or psychological dependence.

"The Problem of Drug Addiction," a chapter from a book written in 1958 by David P. Ausubel, treats the matter as one of social deviance, psychologically speaking. Basically, Dr. Ausubel approves of the official condemnation of illicit drugs in this country, and his discussion is a persuasive statement of that position. His views, rejected in some quarters, reflect the general attitude that has prevailed in this century.

The second selection concentrates on drug use among college students, but much of what Helen H. Nowlis says is true of high school students as well. In "The Student and His Culture," she looks sympathetically at the problems confronting college students, their discontent with their world as they find it, and the temptation to use drugs—specifically LSD—that often arises. Although the attraction and use of LSD have declined since the original publication of her report, Dr. Nowlis' analysis of student motivation remains valid and may be applied to other campus drug patterns.

Dr. Andrew Weil approaches drugs from an altogether different angle in his book *The Natural Mind*. He sees the desire to "get high" not as a problem, either social or individual, but rather as a basic human instinct to alter con-

sciousness. The problem stems from responses to and attempts to repress this basic drive, he contends in "Why
People Take Drugs," the third and last excerpt in this
section.

THE PROBLEM OF DRUG ADDICTION [1]

The Meaning of Drug Addiction

It is necessary at the outset to define what we mean by
the terms, *drug addiction* and *addicting drugs*. According to
traditional medical usage, addiction refers to a condition
brought about by the repeated administration of *any* drug
"such that continued use of the drug is necessary to maintain
normal physiological function, and discontinuance of the
drug results in definite physical and mental symptoms." But
usually, when the term *drug addiction* is used without further qualification, addiction to the opiate group of narcotic
drugs is meant.

It has also been customary to distinguish between drugs
that are habit-forming and drugs that are addicting. The
former group of drugs are said to induce "a condition in
which the habitué desires a drug but suffers no ill effects
on its discontinuance." Thus, the drugs in tobacco, coffee,
cola drinks, and laxatives are frequently characterized as
habit-forming but not as addicting. The present writer, however, fails to perceive any value in this distinction. Physical
or psychological habituation, after all, best describes the condition that develops during the course of drug addiction and
which is responsible for the mental and physical symptoms
that arise when the drug is discontinued. Furthermore, many
habitual users of tobacco, coffee, alcohol, and laxatives experience profound physical or psychological discomfort
when they voluntarily or otherwise forgo their usage. Hence,

[1] From *Drug Addiction: Physiological, Psychological, and Sociological Aspects*,
by David P. Ausubel, M.D., member, Bureau of Educational Research, University
of Illinois, and author of many articles on drug addiction. Random House. '58.
p 9-15. Copyright © 1958 by Random House, Inc. Reprinted by permission of
the publisher.

it would be quite correct to use the terms habit-forming and addicting synonymously and to refer to common habit-forming drugs as addictive in nature.

It is true, however, that although opiates and tobacco are both addicting or habit-forming drugs, addiction to opiates is *in addition* characterized by a phenomenon that does not occur in relation to tobacco or coffee. Habitual usage of an opiate results in physiological changes within the tissues of the body that invariably bring about a stereotyped pattern of physical symptoms when the drug is withdrawn. This phenomenon of physical dependence is responsible for the fact that discontinuance of opiates in addicted persons results in more serious and invariable physical distress than is the case when tobacco or coffee are similarly withdrawn. Furthermore, in the latter instances, since tissue changes are not involved, the symptoms of withdrawal are quite variable and are largely or completely absent in many individuals. We can conclude, therefore, that drugs can be habit-forming or addicting even though physical dependence is not involved. But if physical dependence also occurs, the type of addiction that results is characterized by more severe and invariable physical symptoms when the drug is withdrawn.

Thus, when we ask to what drugs can one become addicted, we must include a large number of drugs—stimulants such as cocaine, Benzedrine, and mescaline; depressants such as marijuana, opiates, and their derivatives; hypnotics and sedatives such as bromides and barbiturates; and alcohol, tobacco, caffeine, and certain kinds of laxatives. Physical dependence, however, is a relatively rare phenomenon in the total picture of drug addiction. True physical dependence probably only develops in relation to opiate and opiate-like drugs, although characteristic withdrawal symptoms are sometimes found in chronic alcoholism and invariably in advanced cases of barbiturate addiction. Nevertheless, as will be pointed out later, physical dependence is by no means the most important or most dangerous aspect of drug addic-

tion. When it does take place it merely guarantees the
occurrence of a relatively severe and invariable group of
withdrawal symptoms. The actual prognosis of a case of drug
addiction, however, is primarily a function of psychological
and personality factors.

Ways in Which Drug Addiction Is Harmful

Drug addiction is merely a descriptive term, defining a
state of habituation brought about by the continued use of
certain drugs. In and of itself it carries no evaluative conno-
tations. It is harmful or undesirable only if it occurs under
conditions which are detrimental to individual or social welfare. Like any other commodity or habit, drugs and habituation to drugs may be used for good or for evil, and can be
considered good, bad, or indifferent in value only in terms
of their effects. If the compulsive use of various drugs
results in unnecessary physical damage, loss of psychological
efficiency, or in social disorganization, addiction is harmful.
But contrary to common belief, the mere fact that a drug
is habit-forming or is used habitually does not necessarily
stamp the drug or the habit as vicious or sinister. This
information merely informs us that special care is required
in the use of the drug, since the dangers of abuse are naturally enhanced if such abuse may become habitual.

Several examples may help to clarify this point. A great
number of individuals who have visual defects, missing
teeth, or amputated limbs become habituated to the use of
eyeglasses, dentures, or prosthetic devices. Although these
artificial aids soon become absolutely essential for adequate
vision, chewing, or locomotion, few persons would regard
such habituation as harmful. Similarly, it makes good sense
to relieve the pain of incurable cancer with addicting anal-
gesics and to sometimes administer habit-forming hypnotics
to certain individuals suffering from chronic insomnia. These
latter decisions, naturally, can only be made by competent
medical specialists. And insofar as the moderate use of coffee,
alcohol, and tobacco has not been demonstrated to be in-

jurious, the addictive aspects of such practices need not be viewed with alarm [from the medical point of view].

On the other hand, habituation is harmful and undesirable: if it leads unnecessarily to loss of natural functional capacities; if addicting drugs are used for mild and transitory disorders when other less extreme and nonaddicting remedies would suffice; and, lastly but most important, if the effects of such addiction are injurious to the individual or to society. Thus, it is definitely unwise to use routinely, over protracted periods of time, habit-forming laxatives and hypnotics for mild and self-limited cases of constipation and insomnia respectively. It is obviously even more indefensible to become habituated to drugs that may readily impair physical and mental health or result in widespread social disorganization when no medical indications whatsoever exist for their use.

Need for Social Regulation of Opiate Use

Society's right to suppress opiate addiction is predicated upon two very different kinds of propositions. The first kind of proposition, which merely asserts that such addiction is harmful to both the individual and to society, can be empirically tested. The second kind of proposition, however, is based entirely on a philosophy of law or government and cannot be either proven or disproven. This proposition rests on the assumption that society may invade the domain of personal rights both to protect the general welfare and to prevent the individual from knowingly or unknowingly inflicting harm upon himself. Although unprovable, this latter proposition is so firmly embedded in our entire legal system and structure of government that it requires no further justification.

Interestingly enough, the drug addict generally tends to reject both sets of propositions. In the same breath he denies that opiate addiction is injurious to the individual or to the social order, and belligerently asserts that, even if it were, an individual's vices are his own private affair. According to him, opiates are no more of a social menace than alcohol or tobacco. Hence he sees no reason why he should be forbidden the enjoyment of his special brand of drug pleasure when other persons are at liberty to do as they please with respect to their drugs. He maintains that if he were assured a steady supply of drugs and could be spared the time, effort, and concern that normally go into their acquisition, he would experience no difficulty in holding down a job and would even work more effectively under their influence. He proudly points to the alleged existence of a group of brilliant men who are addicts unknown to society and maintain themselves on small daily doses. Finally, he claims that restrictive narcotic laws have caused more addiction than any other single factor.

What are the facts in the case? In the first place, it has been unequivocally established by systematic observation under controlled conditions that when an addict is permitted to use as much drug as he wants, he characteristically becomes lethargic, slovenly, undependable, and devoid of ambition. The drug-satiated addict loses all desire for socially productive work and exhibits little interest in food, sex, companionship, family ties, or recreation. The so-called push which he attributes to the influence of the drug becomes evident only when he becomes concerned about the source of his next dose. His belief that he can work more efficiently under the influence of drugs is merely an illusion created by the euphoria he experiences with drug usage. Objective tests actually demonstrate deceleration in speed of tapping and learning and in verbal and motor reaction time. The typical addict uses as high a dose of the drug as he can afford or obtain, and almost invariably more than he requires to remain free of the uncomfortable symptoms he experiences upon withdrawal of the drug. Hence the brilliant surgeon or philosopher addict who limits himself to a small dose to "steady his nerves" or "sharpen his mental faculties" is mostly a myth.

These pernicious effects of narcotic addiction on individual productivity are hardly surprising in view of the known adjusive properties of opiates for addiction-prone individuals [as reported in a medical journal]. If "the goal of personal satisfaction" normally achieved through socially valuable activities directed toward "security, prestige, family attachments, financial independence . . . can be acquired through the simple expedient of injecting morphine, these activities are rendered superfluous, and the addict becomes a useless burden on his family and society in general." Primarily for this reason, society, for its own protection, is required to legislate against drug addiction. "Easy availability [the report goes on to say] would lead to . . . use by thousands or perhaps hundreds of thousands of neurotic, psychopathic or otherwise inadequate people of whom there are plenty in society."

In times of social demoralization [the writer himself has written in a journal of psychiatry] the habit, because of its efficient adjusive value, would be acquired by a large segment of the population; and as shown by historical experience in China and Egypt would be a major contributing factor toward perpetuating poverty, ignorance, and lack of social and economic progress.

Although the writer certainly holds no brief for the intemperate use of alcohol, it is important to recognize that alcohol is a decidedly less dangerous drug. It does not generate sufficient euphoria and its adjusive value is insufficient to serve as a complete and satisfactory substitute for all productive human activity. The acquisition of genuine tolerance to the effects of alcohol, and hence, the acquisition of true physical dependence based on such tolerance, is relatively rare. It is true that alcoholism is currently responsible for more illness, death, crime, and social disorganization than is opiate addiction; but it must be remembered that the number of persons knowingly exposed to narcotics is infinitesimal compared to the number of persons using alcoholic beverages. In any event, the evils associated with excessive use of alcohol provide more of an argument for the control of such abuses than they provide justification for the

elimination of narcotic controls. Despite the addict's statement to the contrary, law enforcement has materially reduced the incidence of drug addiction. The illegality of drug
addiction has incentive value per se only to the aggressive,
antisocial psychopath and to the thrill-seeking adolescent.

It has been convincingly argued that drug addiction, like
alcoholism, is a disease requiring treatment rather than a
crime requiring punishment. . . . This proposition certainly
has considerable merit. It is, at any rate, difficult to appreciate the logic or consistency of regarding the chronic alcoholic as an ill person and the drug addict as a criminal.
There is a marked difference, however, between *not* regarding drug addiction as a crime and legalizing the practice,
that is, allowing everyone free access to the drug. The suggestion advanced by certain well-intentioned but misin-
formed persons that the habit be legalized for present known
addicts only is unsatisfactory, because it would provide legal
and moral sanction for the habit and thus encourage its
spread.

THE STUDENT AND HIS CULTURE [2]

Assuming that it is more profitable to look at the drug
user than at the drug and that most reasonably normal people do not continue to do something that does not provide
them with at least some satisfaction, we now look at the
student and the demands of the world in which he lives
and grows. Such questions as whether using drugs should
be satisfying, or whether the needs they are perceived to
satisfy are legitimate needs, are in some ways irrelevant.
The needs are felt as real, they motivate behavior, and they
cannot be wished away.

Venturing into this area warrants a repeated warning,

[2] From *Drugs on the College Campus*, by Helen H. Nowlis, professor of psychology and research consultant on student affairs, University of Rochester, and
director of a drug education project sponsored by the National Association of
Student Personnel Administrators and the Food and Drug Administration. (Anchor
Books) Doubleday. '69. p 21-31.

lest it be forgotten. Just as students differ, students who use drugs differ, and it is a great mistake to get overenthusiastic about any one explanatory idea. This becomes increasingly true as drug use spreads. There are, however, some general observations which may be useful.

All college students are at one or another stage in growth from childhood to adulthood. This growth process involves both the unlearning of modes of behavior which were appropriate and rewarded in childhood and the learning of new modes in accordance with society's definition of the adult role, a definition which is neither clear nor consistent. Becoming adult involves, at a minimum, substituting independence for dependence, individual identity for borrowed or assigned identity, and meaningful social relationships with a variety of individuals outside the family circle for basic relationships inside the family. It involves development of meaningful sexual identity and appropriate masculine or feminine roles and a meaningful relationship to life and the meaning of life. The attainment of maturity also involves the ability to postpone immediate gratifications in the interest of long-range goals. (The atomic bomb and the "buy-now-pay-later" philosophy seem to have contributed little to the development of this ability in either youth or adult.)

Neither meaningful identity nor a set of values to live by can be bestowed like a mantle. They must become a part of one's being, and the process of internalizing them can be painful, both for the person and for those who care. Becoming independent may, some believe must, involve rebellion. Developing an identity consistent with one's talents and abilities, hopes and dreams, requires hard work and experimentation which may be unsuccessful more often than it is successful. Developing mature, meaningful social relationships is difficult at best and the more so if independence and some degree of identity have not been achieved. Tolerating the frustration involved in postponing gratifications can make other frustrations seem greater. Finding the meaning in life and being at peace with one's self and one's God are goals many adults never attain.

The irony of the appeal of LSD is that, in one way or another, it can be perceived as offering a promise of help in all of these difficult tasks. It seems as if nothing could have been better designed, either by the proponents of LSD or by the mass media which publicized it, to appeal to the personal, social, and emotional needs and the idealism of these young people who are "hung up" in a society which has made adolescence so prolonged and adulthood so uncertain. What LSD is said to offer is inviting fare for the weary traveler, inviting in direct proportion to the degree of weariness.

There are other reasons why students use drugs and, for the most part, they are the same reasons why adults use drugs such as alcohol, tranquilizers, amphetamines, barbiturates, aspirin, nicotine, and caffeine. All of these are widely used by a variety of people for a variety of reasons—for a change of pace, to change mood, to reduce anxiety, for a pick-up, to combat fatigue, to relieve tensions, to relieve boredom, to facilitate social interaction, to sleep, just for fun. It would not be surprising to find that some four-year-old watchers of television could name a specific product for each purpose.

Some adults try these drugs, some react badly or do not find what they are seeking and never try again; some use them occasionally; some use them socially; some use them to escape; some are as dependent, psychologically and in some cases physically, as they would be if their dependence were on an opiate. The main difference is that these substances are socially acceptable and are fairly easily available. Man has used drugs throughout the ages to escape from discomfort and misery. It is interesting to note that in our society misery is a condition familiar not only to the socially and economically depressed but also to those who are in the midst of "success."

There are many other appeals. More young people than

most adults would care to admit are weary of chasing the same carrot at the end of the same stick for fourteen to sixteen years; they dream of getting out of "the rat race" just for a while. Some take a junior year abroad, others do their stint in the military, some take time out for Vista, some keep their noses to the grindstone, hating it to varying degrees, some flunk out though not for lack of ability, some take a marijuana dropout on weekends. LSD invites them to do what some want most to do, with the company of like-minded peers as a bonus, to "solve" their problems, whether these be rebellion or the search for independence, for identity, for satisfying social and personal relationships, for values which are not confused and uncomfortable, or for a meaningful religious experience. To "drop out" the LSD way does not require long arguments with the stockholders —parents, deans, other adults—few of whom seem likely to be persuaded that a moratorium is a positive, constructive, appropriate action at this time and for these reasons. LSD can appear to be a painless way to experiment with dropping out, to escape temporarily into a "bright and shiny world," a world in which people are interested in what really seems to matter, not what should matter, what one is and wants to be, not what he should be.

The response of society to student drug use may foster further use when that response is based on assumptions which seem contradictory or hypocritical to the student. For example, it is widely assumed that when there is no medically approved reason for taking a drug the individual has no right to take it. A further questionable assumption is also made: since the only legitimate use of a drug is in the treatment of illness, anyone who takes a drug is, *ipso facto,* ill—or criminal. The students who reject both assumptions point to alcohol as a potent drug about the use of which society makes completely different assumptions: the individual does have the right to choose to take alcohol for other than medical reasons, and the person who uses alcohol properly is not considered to be ill. They then argue that the attitudes toward alcohol should be extended to include other seemingly nondangerous, nonmedical drugs.

The fact that so many young people are ready to consider just what it is that LSD and the group who use it have to offer should make us think not only about students and drugs but also about the society in which the student has grown up.

The more one inquires into all aspects of the drug problem the more one is impressed with the importance of availability. Has there ever been a society in which drugs were more widely available than in current American society? It is a society dedicated to progress through chemistry. Since infancy the student has learned to open his mouth on command and swallow whatever was popped in to cure what ailed him, and he has watched his parents do the same. A very significant portion of the family budget is often spent on drugs, tobacco, and mood-changing beverages. One study suggests that the average household may have as many as thirty drugs in its medicine cabinet. [R. H.] Blum notes that users of illicit and exotic drugs, in contrast to nonusers, had been ill more often as a child, had been taken to the physician more frequently, and had taken more medications. He also suggests that there are many confirmed "drug optimists," individuals who have grown up confident that for every ill there is a drug which will cure it.

Unfortunately, there are more and more individuals who think that each ill needs not one but many drugs. [C. W.] Wahl has . . . described a symptom complex, "status medicamentosis," which results from indiscriminate medication with too many drugs. He argues that it develops as a result of two social-psychological factors: (1) a widespread and intense belief in the power of medication, a belief which ignores the limitations and side effects of drugs and which is a by-product of constantly hearing about the impressive and diverse successes of medical science, and (2) the deterioration of patient-doctor relationships in an era of increased specialization. Relying more on medication than on the physician, the person medicates himself excessively and indiscriminately. He uses medication as a kind of magical protector and depends on medication rather than people to handle certain emotional drives and needs.

That physicians themselves contribute to this situation is suggested by . . . [Donald Louria in *Nightmare Drugs*]:

At the present time, it is a reasonable estimate that half of the sedatives and tranquilizers prescribed by physicians are given unnecessarily. If the medical profession will rigidly limit the use of these drugs, it is likely that at least some of those who would otherwise illicitly use them would realize the inadvisability of medicating themselves with these potentially dangerous agents.

Another important aspect of current society is its attitude toward risk. Students have grown up in an atmosphere which takes risks for granted and assumes that there is little that can be done without risk. Risk taking ideally involves rational decisions about the utility of a certain action, decisions which are based on informed estimates of both the value of the goal and the probability of gain or loss, of reward or disaster. Despite obvious risks, cars are driven on freeways and airplanes are filled with passengers because rational men continue to believe in the utility of doing so. But risk taking is more often based not on rational decision but on irrational thinking, habit, hunch, impulse, mood, or information that is inadequate and erroneous. A temporary feeling of invulnerability may lead the individual to believe "it won't happen to me." Or feelings of hopelessness or of being discriminated against may lead him to believe he has very little to lose and much to gain. Thus an adequate description of the risks involved in drug use may serve as an effective deterrent to some but have no effect or even the opposite effect on others.

One does not have to look far to see other aspects of the society in which the young person finds himself which may be relevant in understanding much of what is happening. The fact that our society holds certain beliefs to be inviolable even as it violates them adds other complications to the process of growing up. Most young people have learned their verbal lessons well—love not hate, brotherhood not discrimination, equal opportunity, freedom from fear and want, equality in diversity, the basic worth of the individual. But the world is not like that. With the straightforwardness that so often characterizes youth, some scream "hypocrisy" while others set about trying to live according to these basic beliefs.

It has frequently been pointed out that ours is an achievement-oriented, environment-dominating society which almost exclusively values and rewards intellectual or cognitive performance to the exclusion of the life of emotion and feeling. It is a society which often measures success and prestige in terms of material possessions, which considers a young person privileged if he comes from a family which has a modern home, several cars, and income sufficient to provide travel, a college education, membership in a country club, or perhaps a summer home. Far more young people than those who turn to drugs are uneasy in this climate. Some of them look at eminently "successful" parents and do not like what they see or sense. They wonder if getting an education in order to get a job which will provide them with sufficient income to live in the suburbs and be miserable, become alcoholic, develop ulcers, get divorced, is worth the struggle. "There must be something else." The books they read—Sartre, Hesse, Thoreau, Heller, Heinlein, Huxley, Bellows, Tolkien—suggest that there may be.

They feel the need for deep and meaningful experience in an increasingly secular society. Because the church, as organized religion, seems to reflect so many of the trends in society which they find distasteful, they are attracted to the Eastern religions with their emphasis on mysticism and personal religious experience. They want a personally meaningful part in a world which seems so full of aggression, discrimination, poverty, famine, alcoholism, divorce, and hypocrisy that the individual seems superfluous. They want a "frontier" in which to find adventure, challenge, and an opportunity to prove themselves at a time when the only frontiers available for the many would seem to be the technological jungle or the world within. Some of them are rejecting the jungle and withdrawing into the inner world.

The explosion in population and urbanization has contributed to an impersonality in which one's identity is more determined by what one owns, where one lives and works or goes to a college, what one wears, in short, what one appears to be, than it is by what one thinks and feels and is. The explosion in communication, technology, and the mass media has resulted in what . . . [Kenneth Keniston in *Drug Use and Student Values*] . . . has called "stimulus flooding," a constant bombardment of information, of points of view, of advertising, of happenings in every corner of the globe, even in outer space—more information than any man can process, more din than he can tolerate. In perfectly good human fashion he responds by screening it out, ignoring it, protecting himself against more and more of it, and by becoming numb. But the screen may become so dense that it isolates him as well from direct experience with the simple, the beautiful, the unexpected in the world around him. The preoccupation of some of the dropouts with flowers, sunsets, folk songs, togetherness, and meditation is not without significance, nor is the preoccupation of others with a din of their own making. There is more than one way to shut out the world.

WHY PEOPLE TAKE DRUGS [3]

The use of drugs to alter consciousness is nothing new. It has been a feature of human life in all places on the earth and in all ages of history. In fact, to my knowledge, the only people lacking a traditional intoxicant are the Eskimos, who had the misfortune to be unable to grow anything and

[3] From *The Natural Mind*, by Andrew Weil, M.D., writer and researcher on drugs and related questions of altered consciousness. Houghton. '72. p 17-23, 30-8. Copyright © 1972 by Andrew Weil. Reprinted by permission of the publisher Houghton Mifflin Company.

had to wait for white men to bring them alcohol. Alcohol, of course, has always been the most commonly used drug simply because it does not take much effort to discover that the consumption of fermented juices produces interesting variations from ordinary consciousness.

The ubiquity of drug use is so striking that it must represent a basic human appetite. Yet many Americans seem to feel that the contemporary drug scene is something new, something qualitatively different from what has gone before. This attitude is peculiar because all that is really happening is a change in drug preference. There is no evidence that a greater percentage of Americans are taking drugs, only that younger Americans are coming to prefer illegal drugs like marijuana and hallucinogens to alcohol. Therefore, people who insist that everyone is suddenly taking drugs must not see alcohol in the category of drugs. Evidence that this is precisely the case is abundant, and it provides another example of how emotional biases lead us to formulate unhelpful conceptions. Drug taking is bad. We drink alcohol. Therefore alcohol is not a drug. It is, instead, a "pick-me-up," a "thirst quencher," a "social lubricant," "an indispensable accompaniment to fine food," and a variety of other euphemisms. Or, if it is a drug, at least it is not one of those bad drugs that the hippies use.

This attitude is quite prevalent in the adult population of America, and it is an unhelpful formulation for several reasons. In the first place, alcohol is very much a drug by any criterion and causes significant alterations of nervous functioning regardless of what euphemistic guise it appears in. In fact, . . . of all the drugs being used in our society, alcohol has the strongest claim to the label *drug* in view of the prominence of its long-term physical effects. In addition, thinking of alcohol as something other than a drug leads us to frame wrong hypotheses about what is going on in America. We are spending much time, money, and intellectual energy trying to find out why people are taking drugs, but, in fact, what we are doing is trying to find out why some people are taking some drugs that we disapprove of. No useful answers can come out of that sort of inquiry; the question is improperly phrased.

Of course, many theories have been put forward. People are taking drugs to escape, to rebel against parents and other authorities, in response to tensions over foreign wars or domestic crises, in imitation of their elders, and so on and so on. No doubt, these considerations do operate on some level (for instance, they may shape the forms of illegal drug use by young people), but they are totally inadequate to explain the universality of drug use by human beings. To come up with a valid explanation, we simply must suspend our value judgments about kinds of drugs and admit (however painful it might be) that the glass of beer on a hot afternoon and the bottle of wine with a fine meal are no different in kind from the joint of marijuana or the snort of cocaine; nor is the evening devoted to cocktails essentially different from the day devoted to mescaline. All are examples of the same phenomenon: the use of chemical agents to induce alterations in consciousness. What is the meaning of this universal phenomenon?

It is my belief that the desire to alter consciousness periodically is an innate, normal drive analogous to hunger or the sexual drive. Note that I do not say "desire to alter consciousness by means of chemical agents." Drugs are merely one means of satisfying this drive; there are many others, and I will discuss them in due course. In postulating an inborn drive of this sort, I am not advancing a proposition to be proved or disproved but simply a model to be tried out for usefulness in simplifying our understanding of our observations. The model I propose is consistent with observable evidence. In particular, the omnipresence of the phenomenon argues that we are dealing not with something socially or culturally based but rather with a biological characteristic of the species. Furthermore, the need for periods of nonordinary consciousness begins to be expressed at ages far too young for it to have much to do with social conditioning. Anyone who watches very young children without revealing his presence will find them regularly practicing techniques that induce striking changes in mental states. Three- and four-year-olds, for example, commonly whirl themselves into vertiginous stupors. They hyperventilate and have other children squeeze them around the chest until they faint. They also choke each other to produce loss of consciousness.

To my knowledge these practices appear spontaneously among children of all societies, and I suspect they have done so throughout history as well. It is most interesting that children quickly learn to keep this sort of play out of sight of grownups, who instinctively try to stop them. The sight of a child being throttled into unconsciousness scares the parent, but the child seems to have a wonderful time; at least, he goes right off and does it again. Psychologists have paid remarkably little attention to these activities of all children. Some Freudians have noted them and called them "sexual equivalents," suggesting that they are somehow related to the experience of orgasm. But merely labeling a phenomenon does not automatically increase our ability to describe, predict, or influence it; besides, our understanding of sexual experience is too primitive to help us much.

Growing children engage in extensive experimentation with mental states, usually in the direction of loss of waking consciousness. Many of them discover that the transition zone between waking and sleep offers many possibilities for unusual sensations, such as hallucinations and out-of-the-body experiences, and they look forward to this period each night. (And yet, falling asleep becomes suddenly frightening at a later age, possibly when the ego sense has developed more fully. We will return to this point in a moment.) It is only a matter of time before children find out that similar experiences may be obtained chemically; many of them learn it before the age of five. The most common route to this knowledge is the discovery that inhalation of the fumes of volatile solvents in household products induces experiences similar to those caused by whirling or fainting. An alternate route is introduction to general anesthesia in connection with a childhood operation—an experience that invariably becomes one of the most vivid early memories.

By the time most American children enter school they have already explored a variety of altered states of consciousness and usually know that chemical substances are one doorway to this fascinating realm. They also know that it is a forbidden realm in that grownups will always attempt to stop them from going there if they catch them at it. But, as I have said, the desire to repeat these experiences is not mere whim; it looks like a real drive arising from the neurophysiological structure of the human brain. What, then, happens to it as the child becomes more and more involved in the process of socialization? In most cases, it goes underground. Children learn very quickly that they must pursue antisocial behavior patterns if they wish to continue to alter consciousness regularly. Hence the secret meetings in cloakrooms, garages, and playground corners where they can continue to whirl, choke each other, and, perhaps, sniff cleaning fluids or gasoline.

As the growing child's sense of self is reinforced more and more by parents, school, and society at large, the drive to alter consciousness may go underground in the individual as well. That is, its indulgence becomes a very private matter, much like masturbation. Furthermore, in view of the overwhelming social pressure against such indulgence and the strangeness of the experiences from the point of view of normal, ego-centered consciousness, many children become quite frightened of episodes of nonordinary awareness and very unwilling to admit their occurrence. The development of this kind of fear may account for the change from looking forward to falling asleep to being afraid of it; in many cases it leads to repression of memories of the experiences.

Yet coexisting with these emotional attitudes is always the underlying need to satisfy an inner drive. In this regard, the Freudian analogy to sexual experience seems highly pertinent. Like the cyclic urge to relieve sexual tension (which probably begins to be felt at much lower ages than many think), the urge to suspend ordinary awareness arises spontaneously from within, builds to a peak, finds relief, and dissipates—all in accordance with its own intrinsic rhythm. The form of the appearance and course of this desire is identical to that of sexual desire. And the pleasure, in both cases, arises from relief of accumulated tension. Both experiences are thus self-validating; their worth is obvious in their own terms, and it is not necessary to justify them by reference to anything else. In other words, episodes of sexual release and episodes of suspension of ordinary consciousness feel good; they satisfy an inner need. Why they should feel good is another sort of question, which I will try to answer . . . [later]. In the meantime, it will be useful to keep in mind the analogy between sexual experience and the experience of altered consciousness (and the possibility that the former is a special case of the latter rather than the reverse).

Despite the accompaniment of fear and guilt, experiences of nonordinary consciousness persist into adolescence and adult life, although awareness of them may diminish. If one takes the trouble to ask people if they have ever had strange experiences at the point of falling asleep, many adults will admit to hallucinations and feelings of being out of their bodies. Significantly, most will do this with a great sense of relief at being able to tell someone else about it and at learning that such experiences do not mark them as psychologically disturbed. One woman who listened to a lecture I gave came up to me afterward and said, "I never knew other people had things like that. You don't know how much better I feel." The fear and guilt that reveal themselves in statements of this sort doubtless develop at early ages and probably are the source of the very social attitudes that engender more fear and guilt in the next generation. The process is curiously circular and self-perpetuating.

There is one more step in the development of adult attitudes toward consciousness alteration. At some point (rather late, I suspect), children learn that social support exists for one method of doing it—namely, the use of alcohol—and that if they are patient, they will be allowed to try it. Until recently, most persons who reached adulthood in our society were content to drink alcohol if they wished to continue to have experiences of this sort by means of chemicals. Now, however, many young people are discovering that other chemicals may be preferable. After all, this is what drug users themselves say: that certain illegal substances give better highs than alcohol. This is a serious claim, worthy of serious consideration. . . .

Now when I say that people take drugs in response to an innate drive to alter consciousness, I do not make any judgment about the taking of drugs. The drive itself must not be equated with the forms of its expression. Clearly, much drug taking in our country is negative in the sense that it is ultimately destructive to the individual and therefore to society. But this obvious fact says nothing about the intrinsic goodness or badness of altered states of consciousness or the need to experience them. Given the negativity of much drug use, it seems to me there are two possibilities to consider: (1) altered states of consciousness are inherently undesirable (in which case, presumably, the drive to experience them should be thwarted); or (2) altered states of consciousness are neither desirable nor undesirable of themselves but can take bad forms (in which case the drive to experience them should be channeled in some "proper" direction). Do we have enough evidence to make an intelligent choice between these possibilities?

Primarily, we need more information about altered states of consciousness. Altered from what? is a good first question. The answer is: from ordinary waking consciousness, which is "normal" only in the strict sense of "statistically most frequent"; there is no connotation of "good," "worthwhile," or "healthy." Sleep and daydreaming are examples of altered states of consciousness, as are trance, hypnosis, meditation, general anesthesia, delirium, psychosis, mystic rapture, and the various chemical "highs." If we turn to psychology or medicine for an understanding of these states, we encounter a curious problem. Western scientists who study the mind tend to study the objective correlates of consciousness rather than consciousness itself. In fact, because consciousness is nonmaterial, there has been great reluctance to accord it the reality of a laboratory phenomenon; psychologists, therefore, do not study consciousness directly, only indirectly, as by monitoring the physiological responses or brain waves of a person in a hypnotic trance or in meditation. Nonmaterial things are considered inaccessible to direct investigation if not altogether unreal. Consequently, there has been no serious attempt to study altered states of consciousness as such.

In the East, psychological science has taken a very different turn. Subjective states are considered more directly available for investigation than objective phenomena, which, after all, can only be perceived through our subjective states. Accordingly, an experiential science of consciousness has developed in the Orient, of which yoga is a magnificent example. It is a science as brilliantly articulated as Western conceptions of neurophysiology, but no attempt has been made to correlate it carefully with the physical realities of the nervous system as demonstrated by the West.

Therefore, Eastern science should be helpful in understanding altered states of consciousness, but it must always be checked against empirical knowledge of the objective nervous system. Now one of the puzzling and unifying features of altered states of consciousness is their relative absence of physical correlates. For example, there are really no significant physiological differences between a hypnotized person and an unhypnotized person, or even any way of telling them apart if the hypnotized subject is given appropriate suggestions for his behavior. As we shall see, the same holds true for the person high on marijuana—he is not readily distinguishable from one who is not high. Consequently, research as we know it in the West really cannot

get much of a foothold in this area, and the scientific literature is dreadfully inadequate.

Nevertheless, I think it is possible to come to some useful
conclusions about altered states of consciousness from what
we can observe in ourselves and others. An immediate suggestion is that these states form some sort of continuum in
view of how much they have in common with each other.
For example, trance, whether spontaneous or induced by a
hypnotist, is simply an extension of the daydreaming state
in which awareness is focused and, often, directed inward
rather than outward. Except for its voluntary and purposeful character, meditation is not easily distinguished from
trance. Masters of meditation in Zen Buddhism warn their
students to ignore *makyo,* sensory distortions that frequently
resemble the visions of mystics or the hallucinations of schiz-
ophrenics. In other words, there is much cross-phenomenol-
ogy among these states of consciousness, and, interestingly
enough, being high on drugs has many of these same
features, regardless of what drug induces the high.

The sense of physical lightness and timelessness so often
reported by drug users is quite common in trance, meditation, and mystic rapture, for instance. Great ease of access
to unconscious memories is also common in these states.
Hypnotic subjects capable of sustaining deep trances can
be "age regressed"—for example, made to reexperience
their tenth birthday party. In deepest trances, awareness of
present reality is obliterated, and the subject is amnesic for
the experience when he returns to normal consciousness.
In lighter trances, age-regressed subjects often have a sense
of dual reality—the simultaneous experience of reliving the
tenth birthday party while also sitting with the hypnotist.
Exactly the same experience is commonly reported by users
of marijuana, who often find themselves spontaneously reliving unconscious memories as present realities. . . .

I want to underline the idea that these states form a continuum beginning in familiar territory. When we watch a

movie and become oblivious to everything except the screen, we are in a light trance, in which the scope of our awareness has diminished but the intensity of it has increased. In the Oriental scientific literature, analogies are often drawn between consciousness and light: intensity increases as scope decreases. In simple forms of concentration like movie watching or daydreaming, we do not become aware of the power of focused awareness, but we are doing nothing qualitatively different from persons in states of much more intensely focused consciousness where unusual phenomena are the rule. For example, total anesthesia sufficient for major surgery can occur in deep trance; what appears to happen is that the scope of awareness diminishes so much that the pain arising from the body falls outside it. The conscious experience of this state is that "the pain is there but it's happening to someone else." I have myself seen a woman have a baby by Caesarian section with no medication; hypnosis alone was used to induce anesthesia, and she remained conscious, alert, in no discomfort throughout the operation.

I have also seen yogis demonstrate kinds of control of their involuntary nervous systems that my medical education led me to believe were impossible. One that I met could make his heart go into an irregular pattern of beating called fibrillation at will and stop it at will. Such men ascribe their successes in this area solely to powers of concentration developed during regular periods of meditation. There is no need, I think, to point out the tremendous implications of these observations. Because we are unable to modify consciously the operations of a major division of our nervous system (the autonomic system), we are prey to many kinds of illnesses we can do nothing much about (cardiovascular diseases, for example). The possibility that one can learn to influence directly such "involuntary" functions as heart rate, blood pressure, blood flow to internal organs, endocrine secretions, and perhaps even cellular processes by conscious use of the autonomic nervous system is the most exciting frontier of modern medicine. If, by meditation, a man can learn to regulate blood flow to his skin (I have seen a yogi produce a ten-degree-Fahrenheit temperature difference between right and left hands within one minute of getting a signal; the warmer hand was engorged with blood and dark red, the cooler hand was pale), there is no reason why he could not also learn to shut off blood flow to a tumor in his body and thus kill it. . . .

It is noteworthy that most of the world's highest religious and philosophic thought originated in altered states of consciousness in individuals (Gautama [the Buddha], Paul, Mohammed, etc.). It is also noteworthy that creative genius has long been observed to correlate with psychosis and that intuitive genius is often associated with daydreaming, meditation, dreaming, and other nonordinary modes of consciousness.

What conclusions can we draw from all this information? At the least, it would seem, altered states of consciousness have great potential for strongly positive psychic development. They appear to be the ways to more effective and fuller use of the nervous system, to development of creative and intellectual faculties, and to attainment of certain kinds of thought that have been deemed exalted by all who have experienced them.

So there is much logic in our being born with a drive to experiment with other ways of experiencing our perceptions, in particular to get away periodically from ordinary, ego-centered consciousness. It may even be a key factor in the present evolution of the human nervous system. But our immediate concern is the anxiety certain expressions of this drive are provoking in our own land, and we are trying to decide what to make of altered states of consciousness. Clearly, they are potentially valuable to us, not inherently undesirable as in our first hypothesis. They are also not abnormal in that they grade into states all of us have experienced. Therefore, to attempt to thwart this drive would probably be impossible and might be dangerous. True, it exposes the organism to certain risks, but ultimately it can confer psychic superiority. To try to thwart its expression in individuals and in society might be psychologically crippling for people and evolutionarily suicidal for the species. I would not want to see us tamper with something so closely related to our curiosity, our creativity, our intuition, and our highest aspirations.

If the drive to alter consciousness is potentially valuable and the states of altered consciousness are potentially valuable, then something must be channeling that drive in wrong directions for it to have negative manifestations in our society. By the way, I do not equate all drug taking with negative manifestations of the drive to alter consciousness. Drug use becomes negative or abusive only when it poses a serious threat to health or to social or psychological functioning. Failure to distinguish drug use from drug abuse—another unhelpful conception arising from emotional bias —has become quite popular, especially in Federal Government propaganda. The National Institute of Mental Health continues to label every person who smokes marijuana an abuser of the drug, thus creating an insoluble marijuana problem of enormous proportions. Professional legal and medical groups also contribute to this way of thinking. In fact, the American Medical Association has gone so far as to define drug abuse as any use of a "drug of abuse" without professional supervision—an illustration of the peculiar logic necessary to justify conceptions based on emotional rather than rational considerations.

Certainly, much drug use is undesirable, despite the claims of drug enthusiasts, although this problem seems to me much less disturbing than the loss to individuals and to society of the potential benefits of consciousness alteration in positive directions. . . . Our inquiry . . . is directed to the question of why people take drugs. I have tried to demonstrate that people take drugs because they are means of satisfying an inner need for experiencing other modes of consciousness and that whether the drugs are legal or illegal is an unimportant consideration. To answer the question most succinctly: people take drugs because they work.

Or, at least, they seem to.

II. LEGAL ASPECTS OF DRUGS

EDITORS' INTRODUCTION

This section deals with governmental control of, or efforts to control, drug use, abuse, and traffic.

First, there is a brief account of the beginnings of Federal control of illicit drugs, early in the twentieth century. Next, "Today's Drug Laws" discusses the confusion surrounding the use of criminal sanctions to discourage illicit drug taking. The confusion, according to the authors of this extract, a chapter from their book *Drugs and the Public,* arises from the stated dual purpose of harsh legal penalties: public safety and personal health—two considerations that often run counter to each other. And the chief unstated use of law enforcement—as a strong expression of moral disapproval of a deviant minority by the major part of society—further complicates the matter.

In "The Dynamics of Narcotic Control," David F. Musto writes that the main purpose of narcotic control in this country is not moral but political. Specifically, he points out, certain drugs have been related, in the American public awareness, either to ethnic or racial minorities within our borders or to our relations with other countries; as fear of (and hostility toward) different groups has risen and fallen during this century, our official attitude towards drugs has likewise altered.

The report issued in 1973 by the National Commission on Marijuana and Drug Abuse suggested considerable changes at the Federal level in the entire approach to drug use and addiction. It remains to be seen whether any of the report's recommendations will be implemented. In fact, as a Chicago *Sun-Times* account of FBI crime statistics reveals, marijuana arrests in 1973 were 43 percent higher than in 1972. The decriminalization—or, preferably, legalization—

of marijuana is dealt with by the New York *Times* columnist William Safire.

Another legal issue is the question of Federal involvement in and regulation of medical prescription drugs. The last article in the section deals with several aspects of this subject.

EARLY DRUG LEGISLATION[1]

A major step forward in the control of opiate addiction was taken in 1906, when Congress passed the first Pure Food and Drug Act despite opposition from the patent-medicine interests. The pressures to pass the act were intense—generated by Dr. Harvey W. Wiley and his crusading journalistic followers, notably Samuel Hopkins Adams, who were known as "muckrakers." [Samuel Hopkins Adams, *The Great American Fraud: Articles on the Nostrum Evil and Quackery,* reprinted from *Collier's* (1905, 1906, 1907, 1912) by American Medical Association, 1913.]

The 1906 act required that medicines containing opiates and certain other drugs must say so on their labels. [Charles E. Terry and Mildred Pellens, *The Opium Problem* (New York: Committee on Drug Addictions, Bureau of Social Hygiene, Inc., 1928), p. 75.] Later amendments to the act also required that the quantity of each drug be truly stated on the label, and that the drugs meet official standards of identity and purity. Thus, for a time the act actually served to safeguard addicts.

The efforts leading to the 1906 act, the act itself and subsequent amendments, and educational campaigns urging families not to use patent medicines containing opiates, no doubt helped curb the making of new addicts. Indeed, there

[1] From *Licit and Illicit Drugs: The Consumers Union Report on Narcotics, Stimulants, Depressants, Inhalants, Hallucinogens, and Marijuana—Including Caffeine, Nicotine, and Alcohol,* by Edward M. Brecher and the Editors of *Consumer Reports.* Little. '72. p 47. Copyright © 1972 by Consumers Union of United States, Inc. Reprinted by permission of Little, Brown and Co. Mr. Brecher, a writer on health and consumer topics, has received an Albert Lasker Medical Journalism Award.

is evidence of a modest decline in opiate addiction from the peak in the 1890s until 1914. [See, for example, Lawrence Kolb and A. G. Du Mez, *The Prevalence and Trend of Drug Addiction in the United States and Factors Influencing It,* Treasury Department, U.S. Public Health Service, Reprint No 924 (Washington, D.C.: U.S. Government Printing Office, 1924), p. 14, Table 2.]

For those already addicted, however, the protection afforded by the 1906 act and by subsequent amendments was short-lived, for in 1914 Congress passed the Harrison Narcotic Act, which cut off altogether the supply of legal opiates to addicts. As a result, the door was opened wide to adulterated, contaminated, and misbranded black-market narcotics of all kinds. The heroin available on the street in the United States today, for example, is a highly dangerous mixture of small amounts of heroin with large and varying amounts of adulterants. The black market similarly distributes today large quantities of adulterated, contaminated, and misbranded LSD and other drugs. The withdrawal of the protection of the food-and-drug laws from the users of illicit drugs, as we shall show, has been one of the significant factors in reducing addicts to their present miserable status, and in making drug use so damaging today.

TODAY'S DRUG LAWS [2]

Since the early twentieth century Americans have relied on criminal sanctions to stop drug use. Reliance on the law, however, has not stopped drug use nor drug-related harm, but has provoked controversy and impeded efforts to deal with drug misuse.

The confusion and controversy surrounding the law are the result of a conflict, as yet unresolved, between using the

[2] Excerpts from Chapter 6 of *Drugs and the Public,* by Norman E. Zinberg, M.D., associate professor of clinical psychiatry, Harvard Medical School, and John A. Robertson, member of the faculty, Harvard Law School. Simon and Schuster. '72. p 164-200. Copyright © 1972 by Norman E. Zinberg and John A. Robertson. Reprinted by permission of Simon and Schuster.

law to protect order and health and using it to express a moral judgment. Laws are enacted to protect health, safety, and order by penalizing harmful conduct. We usually think of drug laws in this vein. Without penalties to deter drug use, it is thought that crime, violence, personal injury and eventually social chaos will occur. Accompanying this goal is one with a decidedly moralistic bent: all drug use, whatever its consequences, is wrong. Criminalizing drug use thus reinforces moral feelings and protects a moral code increasingly under attack.

As long as the law hovers between the goals of morality and utility, the law will foment controversy without lessening the damage of harmful drug use. The two goals are often incompatible. The first, that of treating and rehabilitating drug users, may recognize that some drug use harms no one or even is functional for the user, and thus contradicts the criminal treatment on which the second depends. In attempting to achieve both aims, one or the other inevitably suffers. With the present laws the desire to condemn and punish has taken precedence over the need to treat. Drug use is thus more damaging than a regime concerned solely with health would allow, and as a further consequence, the drug laws engender conflict, rather than consensus, about the place of private drug use in modern society.

. . . [It will be shown] that the most controversial features of the drug laws—the ones related to indiscriminate condemnation of all drug use—are least justifiable on grounds of protecting the health and welfare of users or anyone else; . . . the functions that such laws serve [will then be discussed].

The Moralistic Elements of the Drug Laws

Certain features of the drug laws provoke hostility and resistance and bring the law into disrepute; they are central to a system that condemns out of hand all drug use. Yet these features are least justifiable as necessary to protect the health and safety of users or the public. We examine several areas in which the law, while avowing concern with health, has actually tried to condemn all drug use.

Overinclusiveness

A drug policy concerned with preventing harm from drug use would concentrate on those drugs that produce harm, and those instances or patterns of use that actually or are likely to cause harm. The present laws are overinclusive in two ways: they treat all drugs, and all uses of a drug, as if they were equally damaging.

Yet it is well known that the depressant, stimulant, analgesic, hypnotic, hallucinogenic, and tranquilizing agents in illegal use differ vastly from one another in pharmacology, psychic effects, motives for use, and consequences for the user. Use of one drug may seldom be harmful; another may be harmful only in clearly defined circumstances; and to use a third may be courting serious risks.

The laws take no account of the relevant distinctions in potential for harm of various drugs and the circumstances of use. Even where legislative or historical accidents have produced disparate categories, the legal judgment is clear: all private drug use is criminal, whatever its actual effects on the user and others.

The monolithic view has produced some absurd results and given credence to claims that the law is arbitrary. Under existing state and Federal laws a drug is classified as either a "narcotic," a "dangerous," or a "harmful" drug. First came "narcotic," which for years has been a convenient catchall for all drugs of public concern. Today "narcotic" remains in the language and minds of millions of people as the generic term for drugs and drug use. The term was introduced into state law by the Uniform Narcotic Drug Act. In 1928 the FBN [Federal Bureau of Narcotics], working through the Commission on Uniform State Laws (a body of lawyers that drafts and recommends legislation for uniform enactment in each state), drafted the act. The act defined "narcotic" to include the opiates and cocaine. With no convincing evidence of dangers, the commission had decided against including marijuana. It did permit each state the option of including marijuana in its definition of "narcotic." Over the years, forty-eight of the fifty states adopted the uniform act. All defined "narcotic" to include marijuana, as well as a hodge-podge of non-narcotic substances ranging from LSD and amphetamines to airplane glue and paregoric.

The uniform act proscribes a number of transactions involving "narcotic drugs," with the penalty determined by the class of transaction rather than by the drug and its potential for harm. For example, all sales of "narcotics" are subject to the same penalty, without regard for the particular drug sold or the features of the sale. Any exchange of drugs, including gift, is defined as sale. Thus, a doctor relieving an addict's withdrawal symptoms with methadone, a professional heroin importer, an addict selling a five-dollar bag, a student sharing a marijuana cigarette with his roommate, or a woman passing one of her own sleeping pills to her husband are guilty of the same crime and subject to the same penalties. Assuming that each transfer threatens harm to a valid state interest, the degree of harm and the seriousness of the harm vary so greatly that essential distinctions are blurred. Instances of actual harm are overlooked when all are included in a single category.

In recent years some states and the Federal Government passed legislation creating a new category of "harmful" or "dangerous" drugs to deal with drugs that seemed to present problems different from narcotics. Offenses involving these drugs are generally treated more leniently than "narcotic" offenses; and in many cases, an act involving a "dangerous" drug is not criminal, whereas with a "narcotic" it is.

Although this category suggests a differentiation among drugs and their effects, the refinement is hard to substantiate. The logic of different drug classifications has not been consistently followed. Rather than introducing clarity, the new category has more often compounded the confusion and contradictions of the laws. To begin with, a separate class for "dangerous drugs" was largely a historical accident. With the Federal laws, for example, dangerous-drug legislation resulted from the inability to fit the regulated drugs into the framework of narcotic and marijuana tax statutes enacted several decades earlier. Where states have chosen to enact a new category for such drugs as amphetamines and barbiturates, rather than expand the list of "narcotic" drugs (which other states have chosen to do), it appears that the characteristics of their users, mainly middle-aged adults, rather than sensitivity to the inconsistencies of the narcotic label have been the motivating factor. A control scheme attuned to the varying potential for harm would not treat leniently drugs that can be extremely dangerous, while harshly penalizing less dangerous drugs. Amphetamines and barbiturates, for instance, produce tolerance, severe withdrawal syndromes, psychosis, high toxicity, and violent or impaired behavior, yet are treated more leniently than marijuana, which has none of those effects. A further anomaly has been added by putting LSD into the dangerous-drug category, while continuing to regard marijuana as a narcotic.

Under the Drug Abuse Control Amendments of 1965—the first Federal regulation of stimulant, depressant, and psychedelic drugs—personal possession was not even penalized, and unlicensed sale or manufacture was subject to a one-year penalty, while marijuana and heroin received mandatory minimum sentences of five years. Such disparities confused even the Federal drug police. In 1968 they testified before Congress that differential treatment increased their problems. Congress attempted to rectify the anomaly by increasing the penalty for sale of dangerous drugs to two years and imposing a maximum penalty of one year in jail for personal possession. Yet the confusion remains. LSD is still subject to the same treatment as amphetamines and barbiturates, while marijuana, the most widely used and least dangerous of illegal drugs, merits more severe sanctions. As a final flourish, THC, the more potent synthetic of the active ingredients in marijuana, was legally grouped with the dangerous drugs.

Classification schemes based on the relative harm of various drugs has become the current legislative vogue, and is hailed as drug reform both in the United States and in England. The Controlled Substances Act, passed in 1970 and now being urged upon the states by the Justice Department, and its British counterpart, the Misuse of Drugs Bill, classify all regulated drugs in five different groupings under one heading. This is widely thought to be a substantial reform, but it is unlikely to alter the dominant tendency to think of all drug use as an undifferentiated phenomenon. Aside from inconsistencies in the relative rankings of the drugs, the fact that all uses of the regulated drugs, whatever their effects, remain criminal indicates that dealing with damaging drug use is not the sole concern of the law.

Except for overt poisons, it is rare that every use of an illegal drug represents the same degree of danger to everyone. Yet under the law all uses of a drug are proscribed, no matter that the motives for use vary tremendously. Peyote or LSD may be used in religious ceremonies by organized cults or individuals; in carefully controlled settings, by experienced, aware individuals, with expert supervision; or as an adjunct to psychotherapy. It may also be taken in the search for yet another kick by a prepsychotic, a depressed teenager, an adult, or a youth seeking peer group approval. Even opiates, when they are provided regularly, may help people to function and be productive: doctor-addicts, the romantic poets, and the ordinary British addicts are the most obvious examples.

The most basic flaw in a system that penalizes without regard to harm every act of use or possession is its clash with the fundamental safeguard of Anglo-American jurisprudence that only the occurrence and not the potentiality of harm be penalized. The vast majority of criminal statutes act *post facto*—they penalize conduct after it has caused injury. A system whereby an intention to steal, say, was made a crime might, assuming detection of intentions were possible, be an efficient way of preventing theft. Yet the price of such efficiency would be the nightmare of thought control, and the injustice of arresting people who, despite their intention, never actually do steal. Where the law penalizes actions prior to the occurrence of actual harm, as with the crimes of attempt, conspiracy, drunken driving, etc., the law occupies an anomalous position, and . . . is criticized when used too frequently. Such crimes are limited to conduct that is clearly preparatory to, and certain to produce, an undesired harm. With conspiracy, for example, an actual overt act in further-ance of the unlawful design must be shown to have occurred to prove the crime. Nor does one "attempt" murder merely by harboring a desire to kill his wife, buying a gun, and waiting in ambush by the garage as she parks the car. Some further act that shows beyond a doubt the intention and likelihood of its completion is required. Similarly, a high degree of probability that harm will result underpins intoxi-cated-driving statutes. Some may be able to negotiate the road quite ably when intoxicated, but there exists massive evidence that most people cannot. We assume quite reason-ably that drunken driving is likely to produce accidents. In all these instances, no matter how direct the causal chain between conduct and eventual harm may seem, we are ex-tremely hesitant to prohibit an act short of actual harm.

The drug laws ignore these limitations—because, of course, all drug use is generally believed to be harmful in itself and to lead to worse harm. . . .

Because some uses of a drug may be harmful, it does not follow that all uses are, or that every use must be prohibited to avoid those few harmful ones. Prohibition of all use is justified only when the evidence shows that most uses of the drug are likely to be damaging, or that it is impossible to use the drug with discrimination. Even then, it does not automatically ensue that criminal sanctions are the most efficient way of preventing harm from drug use. The vice of the present system is that we approach dangerously close to the penal code of Lewis Carroll's Red Queen, where the virtue of punishing likelihoods and intentions is proclaimed as "all the better," since punishment before the harm obviates the harm that would otherwise have occurred. Total condemnation of all drug use is not necessary if our object is to prevent damage, but it is essential if our real intention is to express a moral judgment.

Punishment

Drug penalties are among the most severe on the books. Only murder, rape, and kidnapping receive equivalent treatment. In many states armed robbery, manslaughter, and a variety of other violent crimes are often treated more leniently than drug selling.

Yet there is no evidence that the extreme penalties actually deter people from using drugs in a damaging way or, indeed, from using drugs at all; and there is growing evidence that excessive penalties cast the law into disrepute. The length of penalties, the practice of punishing a single act as multiple offenses, mandatory minimum sentences, and civil commitment programs are difficult to justify in health terms, but they are readily understandable as the wages of sin.

The length of drug sentences is punitive in a relative and absolute sense. In relation to other social harms—such as violence to people or property, injury or death resulting from automobile accidents, and the high infant mortality rates in the black ghetto—the harm from drug use appears minimal. Usually there is no tangible victim, and self-inflicted harm ranks low in the hierarchy of social interests. Thus, drug sentences are objectionable because frequently nothing has been done deserving retribution; and when there is harm, the Draconian penalties are out of all proportion.

The Federal sentences, until recently, averaged two to five years for simple possession of marijuana and narcotics, five to ten years for first offense of sale or possession for sale, ten to forty for a second sale offense. The Controlled Substances Act, while reducing all possession penalties to one-year imprisonment, created a new category of "dangerous special drug offender," who may receive up to twenty-five years' imprisonment. Persons convicted of a "continuing criminal enterprise," as defined by the act, may receive up to life. New York in 1969 made a life sentence mandatory for possession or sale of more than sixteen ounces of heroin, morphine, cocaine, or opium. Texas allows from one year to life for simple possession of any amount of marijuana. Some states punish sale to a minor of a narcotic (including marijuana) with life imprisonment, and Georgia allows the death penalty. Some states would permit the incarceration for life of a twenty-one-year-old college student who shares a "joint" with his twenty-year-old roommate.

Ancillary drug activities are often treated more strictly than use or possession. Merely being in the company of one possessing narcotics illegally could result in a five-year prison term in Massachusetts, while simple possession draws three. A doctor who treats a drug-dependent patient without notifying state authorities risks several years in jail and loss of his medical license. In some states, removing the label from a prescribed medicine is an offense. Most courts tend to place a broad construction on the prohibited actions. . . . Fleeting possession of minute nonusable quantities of a drug is as criminal as possessing large quantities. While there are factors that often prevent adherence to this rigid schedule, high penalties and jail sentences are imposed often enough to cause serious concern. Although there have been noticeable changes in recent years, judges often think that marijuana is as dangerous as heroin because of their equivalent legal treatment, and they sentence accordingly. In other cases, a well-informed and humane judge will have no discretion at all to tailor the sentence to the particular offender. . . .

Many statutes require a judge to impose a minimum jail term in every case. Discretion to sentence according to the background and character of the defendant and the circumstances of the case has been removed because it is feared that the judge might not be punitive enough toward drug offenders. Congress, in 1952 and 1956, provided mandatory minimum sentences for most drug offenses. Judges were not permitted to suspend sentences or grant probation. The right to parole was also severely limited. They had no choice but to sentence every seller to at least five years in jail, and every user to a prison term.

In actual operation, mandatory minimum sentences have had an opposite effect. Limitation of judicial discretion actually amounts to a transfer of that discretion to the police and prosecutor. Their decision to arrest and prosecute becomes simultaneously a sentencing decision if guilt can be established. It is highly questionable whether the sentencing function should be performed by officials whose role in the criminal process is detecting violations and initiating prosecutions. This undermines the checks and balances built into the system, and gives inordinate weight to the subjective decisions of police and prosecutors. . . .

These features of drug sentences are difficult to support in the absence of evidence that penalties actually do prevent drug use, harmful or otherwise. Legal sanctions, along with drug availability, peer-group pressure, education, and family background, are one of many variables that influence the decision to take a drug. The dismal failure of alcohol prohibition and the current wide use of psychoactive drugs suggest that the threat of punishment is by no means the most significant factor. . . .

Two limitations of criminal sanctions further weaken the power of the law to deter: the chances that the criminal activity will never be detected and, if it is, that no punishment will be imposed. The threat of punishment is an abstraction, lacking substance unless there is a high probability that it will be applied in a particular case. But the drug user knows how improbable is his arrest. He may not even know anyone who has ever been arrested. He knows that nonusers cannot readily detect drug intoxication. He also learns to control his "high" to avoid suspicion by nonusers. He will use the drug only at certain times and places, may not keep a supply on the premises, and refuse to obtain drugs even for friends. But even if he is detected, actual punishment is still highly problematic. At present few marijuana users go to jail. If they are students, middle class, reasonably cooperative, and repentant, the case will probably be continued without a finding and eventually be dismissed if no further drug involvement occurs. At worst, they will be put on probation and given a suspended sentence. . . .

Since 1962 many states have enacted statutes that allow addicts to be committed either civilly or in lieu of punishment to treatment centers for long periods. Yet even here, where the law purports to rehabilitate and treat, in operation it works out as punishment. While hailed as a new departure in drug control and a humane shift from a police approach, these programs are indistinguishable from a frankly punitive approach and, in some cases, are worse. . . .

Cavalier Lawmaking

The legal policy of penalizing all drug use and possession has not resulted from clear and convincing evidence that drug use is damaging, and that the damage can be best prevented by criminal law. Accident, distortion, or disregard of information, and an almost naive acceptance of any charge about the evil of drugs, dominate the lawmaking process. . . .

At different junctures in the history of marijuana control, different claims about the harmful effects of the drug have been put forth to justify legislative action. Upon closer examination, the substance of one claim has evaporated, only to have a new one take its place, and criminal prohibition is maintained.

Federal prohibition of marijuana occurred after three days of congressional hearings in 1937. Howard Becker [in *The Outsiders*] has described how the Federal Bureau of Narcotics under Harry Anslinger created a marijuana problem in the press, drafted the bill, and called the hearings leading to the passage of the Marijuana Tax Act. The chief argument advanced in favor of control was that marijuana produced insanity and led to voilent crime. The Senate report [of hearings before the subcommittee on taxation in 1937] described the danger in these terms:

Under the influence of this drug marijuana the will is destroyed and all power of directing and controlling thought is lost. Inhibitions are released. As a result of these effects, many violent crimes have been committed by persons under the influence of this drug. Not only is marijuana used by hardened criminals to steel them to commit violent crimes, but it is also being placed in the hands of high school children in the form of marijuana cigarettes by unscrupulous peddlers. Its continued use results many times in impotency and insanity.

The method of proving these claims left much to be desired. They quoted hearsay statements of an anecdotal nature, relating incidents of murder or violence that were allegedly the result of marijuana intoxication. One witness, for instance, stated [during the hearings before the House Ways and Means Committee in 1937]: "I believe in some cases that one marijuana cigarette may develop a homicidal maniac probably to kill his brother [sic]."

A study by [John] Kaplan, in *Marijuana: The New Prohibition,* analyzes each report and finds inadequate the evidence that marijuana was the cause. In most cases the source was a newspaper or magazine story in which a police officer or an arrested suspect reported marijuana use before the commission of a violent crime.

The poor quality of the evidence was pointed out to Congress by Dr. William C. Woodward, who had previously participated in an investigation of marijuana with the Commission on Uniform State Laws:

It has surprised me that the facts on which these [newspaper] statements have been made have not been brought before this committee by competent primary evidence. We are referred to newspaper publication concerning the prevalence of marijuana addiction. We are told that the use of marijuana causes crime.

But as yet no one has been produced from the Bureau of Prisons to show the number of prisoners who have been found addicted to the marijuana habit. . . . Informal inquiry shows that the Bureau of Prisons has no evidence on that point.

You have been told that school children are great users of marijuana cigarettes. No one has been summoned from the Children's Bureau to show the nature and extent of the habit among children.

Inquiry of the Children's Bureau shows that they have had no occasion to investigate it and know nothing particularly of it.

Moreover, there is in the Treasury Department itself, the Public Health Service, with its Division of Mental Hygiene. . . . That particular bureau has control at the present time of the narcotics farms that were created about 1929 or 1930 and came into operation a few years later. No one has been summoned from that bureau to give evidence on that point.

Informal inquiry by me indicated that they have had no record of any marijuana or cannabis addicts who have ever been committed to those farms.

The Bureau of the Public Health Service has also a division of pharmacology. If you desire evidence as to the pharmacology of cannabis, that obviously is the place where you can get direct and primary evidence rather than the indirect hearsay evidence.

Congress disregarded Woodward's criticism, dismissed him as an uncooperative witness, and passed the law.

When in the late 1940s it became clear that marijuana was not the monster claimed in 1937, the rationale for prohibition shifted. At the original hearings, Commissioner Anslinger entered into this exchange:

CONGRESSMAN DINGELL: I was just wondering whether the marijuana addict graduates into a heroin . . . user?

ANSLINGER: No, sir; I have not heard of a case of that kind. I think it is an entirely different class. The marijuana user does not go in that direction.

For the first time the link to heroin addiction, previously denied by Anslinger, began to appear as a reason for criminal penalties. There is evidence that the FBN officials switched the main danger of marijuana from instantaneous murder, rape, and insanity to the "schooling it provided future addicts." . . . Again, there was scant evidence for this newfound danger. The FBN was claiming an upsurge in heroin addiction in the postwar period, but there was no way to relate that development to marijuana use, nor could physiological or chemical connection between marijuana use and heroin experimentation be shown. The only proof appeared to be the widely accepted "fact" that most heroin addicts had used marijuana sometime previously to their addiction. The high incidence of opiate addicts of a rural or medical origin belies even that "fact."

In any case, the relevant question is what proportion of marijuana users become addicts, not what proportion of addicts first used marijuana. We would probably find that 100 percent of addicts first used tobacco, alcohol, and even milk, but these are not responsible for heroin addiction. The best statistics on this subject came from California, where marijuana use has grown more rapidly than elsewhere. But these figures show no corresponding rise in heroin addiction. In fact, marijuana use is quite prevalent among both college students and North Africans, two groups with very low rates of opiate addiction. . . .

Advocates of marijuana prohibition still rely on the escalation [to heroin addiction] argument, but they have supplemented it with a new list of dangers, including dangerous driving and psychological dependence. As the focus of attack on the marijuana statutes has shifted from the legislatures to the courts, such claims are increasingly aired. Attacks on marijuana statutes have been mounted on several constitutional grounds, from freedom of religion and privacy to cruel and unusual punishment. In one way or another they at least force courts to apply minimum standards of cogency to the evidence. The results to date suggest that courts are only slightly more rigorous than legislatures in evaluating the alleged dangers of marijuana. In *Commonwealth v. Leis,* the Boston marijuana trial, twenty experts presented evidence on the harm versus the harmlessness of marijuana. Both the lower court and the state supreme court held the marijuana laws to be valid on the ground that the legislature could reasonably think the drug harmful. In its reasoning the higher court demonstrated the power that conjecture and speculation so often exercise over hard fact in dealing with drugs. . . .

The Federal LSD laws, in a curious reversal, also illustrate the ascendancy of emotion over logic and reliable data. The Drug Abuse Control Amendments of 1965 attempted to regulate the manufacture, sale, and distribution of LSD by criminal penalties, but exempted possession of the drug for personal use. Possession penalties were thought to needlessly penalize otherwise law-abiding young people who were experimenting without antisocial tendencies. Fear of arrest might also discourage users from seeking psychiatric aid should they need it. Three years later President Johnson asked and received from Congress a law penalizing personal use and possession of the drug. No new evidence of drug effects had been unearthed in the interim. Use of LSD had, in fact, dwindled in response to rumors that it might cause chromosomal damage. The political need for a tough stand against crime and the unruly activists associated with LSD seems to have been so strong that the lack of firm evidence and the still-relevant arguments of 1965 could be ignored. . . .

Enforcement of Morality

One function of laws against the use and possession of drugs is that they publicly sanction the feeling of most people that drug use is morally wrong, even when no one is hurt. . . . Most people . . . are unable or unwilling to keep law and morality distinct. If drug use is wrong, they reason, it is perfectly natural to have the law express that judgment and punish the immorality when it occurs. Indeed, the need to enshrine moral sentiments in the law often obstructs the desire to lessen the damage from drug use.

Moral entrepreneurs seldom acknowledge their moral aims. Usually they rationalize their goal in terms of public health and order. With drugs, it can be convincingly shown that public health requires controls over distribution and manufacture; but it is less clear that criminalizing personal drug use contributes to that end. In the first place, drugs, except when unavailable, rarely incite crime or violence. While indiscriminate drug use may damage the individual, and by extension consume public resources, most . . . seem able to use drugs without suffering serious damage. Finally, as we have seen, criminal penalties do not deter people, and jailing people is an odd way of helping them.

Even if we assume that the laws are meant primarily to protect a person from his own worst tendencies, the moral import of the law is clear. We tolerate and even encourage riding in airplanes and cars, we overeat, imbibe huge quantities of nicotine and alcohol, climb mountains, sky-dive, and race cars—all at great risk to health, productivity, and the well-being of others. Yet only when personal risk involves drug taking is stern disapproval forthcoming. Such inconsistencies suggest that the drug laws enforce a morality based on the wrongness of private drug use. The code is rooted in indigenous American values and an almost religious view of the nature of man and his place in the universe. According to this code, private, recreational drug use is wrong and must be punished, either because it allows us to achieve undesirable psychic states, or because it is an unacceptable way of achieving otherwise desirable experiences.

In a culture committed to hard work, competition, aggressiveness, sequential thought, and postponed pleasure, the passivity, pleasure, and escape from discursive thought provided by drugs seem wrong. Likewise, where independence and the self-made man are ideals, it seems destructive, or at best unfair, to find happiness, pleasure, and insight artificially, without the industry that usually precedes and lends such states value. The strictness of the standard, which like Victorian sexual mores condemns a single departure, implies a view of man as innately evil. So strong are man's desires, and so vulnerable the wall he erects against his evil instincts, that once the forbidden fruits are tasted, he will fall prey to his appetites. Thus, one shot makes an addict, and one marijuana cigarette often is thought to cause personality disintegration.

The strength of these feelings was evident in the reasoning of the lower court in the *Leis* case, which found marijuana to be harmful because, among other things, it causes "a euphoric and unreal feeling of exhilaration and an abnormally subjective concentration on trivia" and leads "the user to lose perspective and focus his attention on one object to the exclusion of all others." Such reasoning does not spring from a rational assessment of tangible injury to user or others. It rests on a subjective feeling that pleasure, contemplation, and inactivity for their own sake cannot be worthwhile, and are thus wrong. . . .

A Symbol of Power and Prestige

By enforcing a moral judgment about the wrongness of drug use the law also fulfills an important symbolic function. Laws operate both instrumentally and symbolically. In instrumental terms, laws are passed to influence behavior in a direction thought to be desirable. But passage or repeal of a law may also convey a meaning or signification totally unrelated to its instrumental aims. Often the two may conflict, with the unavowed and more powerful symbolic aim taking precedence.

For many years the drug laws have symbolized the limits of socially acceptable conduct and have marked off the deviant from the normal. Recently, with a new type of drug user and growing conflict over the drug laws, the law has come to symbolize more than a moral judgment.

One of the most significant social changes of the past decade is the emergence of youth as a critical social group. Youth, however, have been vociferously sacrilegious in their critique of social institutions. Not only have they aimed their shafts at government, foreign policy, the draft, corporations, and the universities; they have also flagrantly disregarded the sacred cows of traditional sexual and drug morality. Stung by this onslaught of revolutionary rhetoric, idealism and immorality, simultaneously an insult and a threat to their power, the older and more traditionally American social groups have fought back with all the weapons at their disposal. They have more money, power, and access to the political process, and thus have been able to use the lawmaking power to reaffirm the values and prestige damaged by the life-styles of the young. Inevitably the drug laws have been pulled into the conflict; firstly, because drug attitudes and use are sharply age-bound, and secondly, because the drug laws, with their moral implications, symbolize the divergent value systems and life-styles at the heart of the conflict. . . .

Most drug legislation of the past seven years reflects this controversy and, indeed, cannot be understood without reference to the symbolic meaning that enacting or refusing to repeal a drug law conveys. We have described the anomalies in the scope and enactment of LSD legislation. While the case for banning all uses of LSD in health terms is difficult to sustain, the meaning of outlawing its use . . . is not. It states clearly and forthrightly that advocates of chemically induced utopias are deviants with no say in setting social norms. . . . With so many young people waving the banner of legalization, repeal of marijuana-possession laws would also signify a victory for the current out-groups. Such a concession would validate the critique levied by youth against the system, and correspondingly decrease the status and power of the Establishment. It would also remove one club by which the older generation have maintained their moral and political hegemony. This view explains the often irrational opposition to marijuana reform, and the flagrant disregard by lawmakers of the law's social costs. Where legislators have heeded calls for reform, the legal changes have been minimal; changing the penalty from a felony to a misdemeanor makes little practical difference and in no sense departs from the view that marijuana users are deviant. . . .

Conclusion: The Paradox of Legal Change

Using law for functions unrelated to public health is . . . a costly enterprise, and one that snares us in an insoluble dilemma. We are damned if we keep the present laws, yet their symbolic functions prevent us from taking steps in a new direction.

The situation has come about because the law, to fulfill its latent purposes, has focused increasingly on establishing the deviant status of drug use, and less and less on protecting users. The overinclusive, punitive, and other condemnatory features of the law, however, conflict with existing knowledge about drugs and, more importantly, conflict with the practice of millions of users who find drugs to be something less than the monolithic horror defined by the law. Out of this clash has sprung the controversy enveloping drug questions.

A shift in the law's emphasis from punishment to treatment would restore credibility on all sides and return drug use to a social setting in which damaging use could be dealt with effectively. The controversy would simultaneously diminish because, on the one hand, drug use would be officially recognized as a medical-social problem and, on the other, a sensible legal policy would allow the social consensus which the law's current vulnerability prevents.

The dilemma is that the unconscious needs served by the law and aroused by controversy obstruct the reorientation of the law that the interests of health require. The shift from condemnation to treatment requires a lowered commitment to the law's symbolic ends, yet only a reduced concern with the badness of drugs will halt its use as a surrogate. As long as the law makes drug use criminal, latent functions will be served. The legal change that would interfere with the notion of drugs-as-evil and lead to a less symbolic concern with the law is precisely what is needed, but the situation as presently structured does not permit this. Until this dilemma is resolved, the drug problem will remain with us.

THE DYNAMICS OF NARCOTIC CONTROL [3]

American concern with narcotics is more than a medical or legal problem—it is in the fullest sense a political problem. The energy that has given impetus to drug control and prohibition came from profound tensions among socioeconomic groups, ethnic minorities, and generations—as well as the psychological attraction of certain drugs. The form of this control has been shaped by the gradual evolution of constitutional law and the lessening limitation of Federal police powers. The bad results of drug use and the number of drug users have often been exaggerated for partisan advantage. Public demand for action against drug abuse has led to regulative decisions that lack a true regard for the reality of drug use. Relations with foreign nations, often the sources of the drugs, have been a theme in the domestic scene from the beginning of the American antinarcotic movement. Narcotics addiction has proven to be one of the most intractable medical inquiries ever faced by American clinicians and scientists. Disentangling the powerful factors which create the political issue of drug abuse may help put the problem in better perspective.

Fear of narcotics has grown with the awareness of their use. Dr. Holmes [Oliver Wendell Holmes, Sr., of the Harvard Medical School] in 1860 and Dr. Beard [George Beard, a neurologist and psychiatrist] in the 1870s and '80s warned that narcotics abuse was increasing. They based their attacks not only on direct observation but on the open record of import statistics. By 1900 restrictive laws on the state level had been enacted, and reformers began to look to the Federal Government for effective national regulation. Reform-minded leaders of the health professions agreed on the need to eliminate the nonmedical use of narcotics. Those seeking

[3] From *The American Disease*, by David F. Musto, M.D., assistant professor of history and psychiatry at Yale University, Fellow of the Drug Abuse Council, and consultant to the White House Office for Drug Abuse Prevention. Yale University Press. '73. p 244-50. Reprinted by permission.

strict narcotic controls believed that either the need for money to buy drugs or a direct physiological incitement to violence led to crime and immoral behavior. Inordinate pleasure caused by drugs, moreover, was seen to provide youth with a poor foundation for character development, and a resulting loss of independence and productivity.

The most passionate support for legal prohibition of narcotics has been associated with fear of a given drug's effect on a specific minority. Certain drugs were dreaded because they seemed to undermine essential social restrictions which kept these groups under control: cocaine was supposed to enable blacks to withstand bullets which would kill normal persons and to stimulate sexual assault. Fear that smoking opium facilitated sexual contact between Chinese and white Americans was also a factor in its total prohibition. Chicanos in the Southwest were believed to be incited to violence by smoking marijuana. Heroin was linked in the 1920s with a turbulent age group: adolescents in reckless and promiscuous urban gangs. Alcohol was associated with immigrants crowding into large and corrupt cities. In each instance, use of a particular drug was attributed to an identifiable and threatening minority group.

The occasion for legal prohibition of drugs for nonmedical purposes appears to come at a time of social crisis between the drug-linked group and the rest of American society. At the turn of this century, when the battle for political control of freed blacks reached a peak (as shown by the extent of disenfranchisement, lynchings, and the success of segregation policies), cocaine, a drug popular among whites and blacks and in the North as well as the South, was associated with expression of black hostility toward whites. Chinese and opium smoking became linked in the depressions of the late nineteenth century, when Chinese were low-paid competitors for employment, and this connection intensified during the bitter discrimination shown Orientals in the first decade of this century. The attack on marijuana occurred in the 1930s when Chicanos became a distinct and visible unemployed minority. Heroin, claimed to be an important factor in the "crime wave" which followed World War I, was implicated in the 1950s as part of the Communist conspiracy against the United States. A youth culture which attacked traditional values became closely connected with marijuana smoking and the use of other psychedelics. Customary use of a certain drug came to symbolize the difference between that group and the rest of society; eliminating the drug might alleviate social disharmony and preserve old order.

The belief that drug use threatened to disrupt American social structures militated against moves toward drug toleration, such as legalizing drug use for adults, or permitting wide latitude in the prescribing practice of physicians. Even if informed students of drugs such as Dr. Lawrence Kolb, Sr., in the 1920s argued that heroin does not stimulate violence, guardians of public safety did not act upon that information. The convenience of believing that heroin stimulated violence made the conviction hard to abandon. Public response to these minority-linked drugs differed radically from attitudes toward other drugs with similar potential for harm such as the barbiturates.

Narcotics are assumed to cause a large percentage of crime, but the political convenience of this allegation and the surrounding imagery suggest the fear of certain minorities, and make one suspicious of this popular assumption. During the last seventy-five years responsible officials have stated that narcotics caused between 50 and 75 percent of all crimes, especially in large cities like New York. Narcotics have been blamed for a variety of America's ills, from crime waves to social disharmony. Their bad effects have been given as the excuse for repressing certain minorities, as evidence for stopping legal heroin maintenance in 1919, and as evidence for starting legal heroin maintenance in 1972.

Like the speculated percentage of crimes caused by narcotic use and sales, the number of addicts estimated for the nation appears often to have been exaggerated. Peaks of overestimation have come before or at the time of the most repressive measures against narcotic use, as in 1919 when a million or more addicts and five million Parlor Reds were said to threaten the United States. Both groups were the object of severe penalties, although in retrospect both figures appear to have been enormously inflated. Still, the substantial number of addicts in the United States has presented one of the most enduringly difficult aspects of any proposed control program. The size of this population has made control of misuse in maintenance programs difficult. There has been a fair amount of diversion of drugs to the illicit market and some registration of nonaddicts.

In America, control of narcotics could take only a limited number of legislative forms. The lack of broad Federal police powers inhibited the restriction of drug transactions. The division of Federal and state powers in effect permitted widespread and unscrupulous dissemination of untested products and unsafe drugs. When the danger of narcotics came to the attention of popular reform movements and after carefully phrased Federal legislation was at last enacted in 1914 [in the Harrison Act], it took the Supreme Court five years to overcome the apparent obstacle of states' rights. In 1919 the court permitted the Federal Government almost prohibitory power for prevention of most addiction maintenance. The court's majority affirmed the reformers' belief that simple addiction maintenance was intolerable.

Nevertheless, after 1919, severe constitutional strictures continued to mold enforcement of the Harrison Act. Because all professionals (unless convicted of a violation) had to be treated equally under a revenue statute, the Federal Government could not discriminate against careless or unscrupulous physicians and druggists by refusing them a tax stamp or by employing some other fair form of flexible administrative punishment. This lack of legal accommodation to circumstances, the small number of agents, and a bureaucratic reward system which favored a large number of prosecutions led to harassment and intimidation as a prominent mode of

regulation. Because Government agents feared that prece-
dents might prevent indictment of "dope doctors," exceptions to the no-maintenance rule were few. The mutual
suspicion which grew up between agents and physicians inhibited reasonable enforcement of the law. . . .

The Federal narcotic authorities never forgot that theirs
was a narrow path between Federal and states' rights. As late
as 1937 the Treasury Department chose to prohibit marijuana by a separate law because it feared an attack on the
constitutionality of the Harrison Act. In spite of organized
medicine's opposition in the 1920s, and despite several close
Supreme Court decisions, the extreme interpretation placed
on the Harrison Act in 1919 continued to prevail. Why did
the Supreme Court agree that a Federal statute could outlaw
narcotics, when the Constitution itself had to be amended to
outlaw alcohol? One answer to this may be that in the case of
narcotics the consensus was almost absolute; everyone appeared to agree on the evils of these drugs. For alcohol, there
was no such agreement.

Foreign nations have played important roles in the
American perception of its national drug problem. World
War I is the watershed in national self-consciousness vis-à-vis
foreign powers, dividing respectable opinion on the relative
importance of domestic and international causes of narcotics
use in the United States. In the prewar years the United
States displayed confidence in traditional diplomatic methods and the efficacy of international treaties. Prior to the war
and the immediate postwar security crisis, the usual explanation for the American drug appetite rested on characteristics of American culture—the pace of life, the effect of
civilization, wealth which permitted indulgence, and inadequate state and Federal laws which did not protect citizens
from dangerous nostrums and incompetent health professionals.

After World War I, open official criticism of America's
defects was no longer common. Whereas Hamilton Wright
[a physician who represented the United States at interna-

tional opium conferences before World War I] saw international control of narcotics as a solution to America's
indigenous problem and recognized that this nation would
benefit more than others from international altruism, Representative [Stephen Geyer] Porter [of Pennsylvania, who
represented the United States at conferences] in the 1920s
denied any unusual appetite for narcotics in the United
States, blaming our problem on the perfidy and greed of
other nations. [Representative] Richmond Hobson [of Ala-
bama, a former naval officer active in antinarcotic organizations in the 1920s], equally as patriotic, claimed the country
had an immense number of heroin addicts and consequent
crime waves due to the evil influence of other nations. Hobson viewed America as surrounded by other dangerous con-
tinents—South America sent in cocaine; Europe contributed
drugs like heroin and morphine; Asia was the source of
crude opium and smoking opium; Africa produced hashish.
Porter and Hobson sounded one theme: the American problem was caused by foreign nations. The spirit of national
isolation which excluded participation in the League of
Nations extended easily to international narcotic control.
Americans were encouraged to condemn diplomacy as zeal-
ously as they had once sought conferences and commissions.

Projection of blame on foreign nations for domestic evils
harmonized with the ascription of drug use to ethnic minorities. Both the external cause and the internal locus
could be dismissed as un-American. This kind of analysis
avoids the painful and awkward realization that the use of
dangerous drugs may be an integral part of American society. Putting the blame on others also permits more punitive measures to be taken against certain of the culprits.

The history of American narcotic usage and control does
not encourage belief in a simple solution to the long-
standing problem. Reasonable regulation of drug use requires knowledge of physiological and psychological effects,
an understanding of social causes of drug popularity, and an
appreciation of how legal sanctions will actually affect the

use and harmful results of drug ingestion. In the construction of such a policy, recognition of accidental and irrational factors in past drug legislation is essential, although
no ideal program can be simply extrapolated from an
historical study.

Political judgment and values have been paramount in
the establishment of national drug policies. The common-
sense conclusions reached by legislators, high-ranking government bureaucrats, and influential public figures, without
any special or technical knowledge of drug abuse, are likely
to gain acceptance from other national social and political
institutions. Political judgments made in harmony with popular demands for narcotic control (or release from liquor
control) have a proven longevity. Resisting insistent popular
demands is unusual among public officials; considerable political acumen is required to modify prevailing fear and
anger into constructive programs.

As the pressure for political action reaches a climax,
policy options are almost imperceptibly reduced to the few
which have current political viability. The rapid crystalliza-
tion of public policy in 1919–20 illustrates how quickly this
last stage of policy formulation may pass. Dissidents like
Representative [Lester David] Volk [of New York, a physician and lawyer] and Dr. [Ernest Simons] Bishop [a medical
expert on addiction and legislative consultant] continued to
protest, to little effect. Once the national mood had been
settled, any attempt to reopen the painful question met
strong resistance. The 1919 formulation defined a broad
range of issues in narcotic control, and yet the battle was
waged on curiously narrow lines. In the medical profession,
for example, both those for and against the "disease" concept of addiction carried on their dispute over the question
of whether antibodies or antitoxins were produced by morphine administration. The lack of such substances seemed to
prove that addiction must be a mere habit, and that those
who held out for the "disease" concept had unworthy motives. In that period of crisis over narcotic policies fifty years

ago each side was unwilling to compromise and sought to
sweep the adversary from the field.

Today an issue like methadone maintenance may form
the model on which a consensus is reached. This might lead
toward simple toleration, or to prohibition of natural and
synthetic opiates for nonmedical purposes (which would include "mere addiction"). As new generations confront the
narcotic question, the same old fundamental issues continue
to arise. Current debates over heroin maintenance focus on
such basic questions as the effect of heroin on the body and
personality. One almost hears the voice of Dr. Bishop argu-
ing that if an addict is in heroin balance he is a normal
person as regards the effect of the drug, and Captain Hobson
warning that heroin use gradually destroys the brain's higher
centers. After more than half a century since the Harrison
Act's passage one of the few statements about narcotics on
which there is general agreement is that there is no treatment of hard-core addiction which leads to abstinence in
more than a fraction of attempts. The lack of agreement on
other crucial questions and their relative importance is almost total.

Although social and cultural influences are essential ele-
ments in the creation of the American drug problem, it is
quite possible to provide a viable political response to public outcry and at the same time avoid an objective examination of critical issues: the nature of American society; the
psychological vulnerability of addicts; the physiological
effects of drugs; the social impact of drug use. Our society's
blindness to alcohol's destructive effects is an example of
how denial of reality is compatible with a politically comfortable resolution of a controversial drug problem.

We are now at a time when the credibility of previous
solutions is sufficiently low so that some of the unresolved
questions can be raised and again discussed. Gradually, and
not necessarily as the result of formal decisions, the scientific
and political alternatives regarding drug abuse may, as they
have in the past, diminish. As a new workable political

solution evolves the controversy tends to narrow to a few issues. Ideally, public pressure for elimination of the drug problem should not be met with fewer options. Rather the effective translation of knowledge, scientific and historical, should enable the public to avoid oversimplification, and to exert influence based on more national understanding. But only the most determined efforts can prevent closure on drug policy by those two most powerful forces: fatigue and frustration.

TREATMENT, NOT PENALTIES [4]

The National Commission on Marijuana and Drug Abuse [in March 1973] called . . . for a new approach to narcotics addiction of all kinds, emphasizing treatment rather than punishment and stigmatizing only those habits that threaten society.

In its final [481-page] report to President Nixon and Congress, the commission, headed by Raymond P. Shafer, former governor of Pennsylvania, urged again the legalization of possession of marijuana, which it said was not habit-forming and did not promote crime by those who used it.

It also opposed the mandatory minimum jail sentences for drug sellers . . . [advocated by] President Nixon and Governor Rockefeller of New York. . . . The commission contended that such sentences were "counter-productive" and tended to make juries acquit accused pushers rather than apply the harsh penalties. . . .

Among more than one hundred recommendations, the Shafer Commission proposed the following:

Mandatory treatment programs for those charged with possession of any narcotic except marijuana but no punishment more severe than a $500 fine. "For drug-dependent persons," the commission said, "the only legitimate

[4] From "U.S. Drug Study Stresses Treatment, Not Penalties," article by Warren Weaver, Jr., staff writer. New York *Times*. p 1+. Mr. 23, '73. © 1973 by The New York Times Company. Reprinted by permission.

role of the criminal justice system is to function as an entry mechanism into a treatment system."

A moratorium on all drug education programs in the schools until they can be evaluated and made more realistic, and repeal of all state laws requiring drug education courses.

Public acknowledgment by the liquor industry that "compulsive use of alcohol is the most destructive drug-use pattern in this nation" and research by the industry into the relation between drinking and traffic accidents, violent crime and domestic discord.

An end to advertising of "mood-altering drugs"—sedatives, tranquilizers and stimulants—that promise to produce "pleasurable mood alteration" or halt "malaise caused by stress or anxiety."

Creation of a new independent Federal agency to administer all drug policy, absorbing the functions of ten agencies in the Justice, Treasury and Health, Education and Welfare Departments and the White House.

Retention of existing legal controls on the availability of narcotics, placing "the highest possible restrictions" on heroin. Methaqualone, but not barbiturates, would be included in the restricted classification.

Similarity of Problems

Throughout its report, the Shafer Commission emphasized that socially acceptable conduct like drinking liquor and taking psychoactive pills did not pose a problem fundamentally different from that of using heroin and LSD.

"Instead of assuming that mood alteration through some drugs is inherently objectionable, while similar use of others is not," the report said, "the public and its leaders must focus directly on the appropriate role of drug-induced mood alteration.

"It is no longer satisfactory to defend social disapproval

of a particular drug on the ground that it is a 'mind-altering drug' or 'a means of escape.' For so are they all."

The commission suggested that one reason for the increased use of tranquilizers and stimulants was that "many persons have come to regard very real and fundamental emotions and feelings as abnormal, avoidable, socially and personally unacceptable and, worst of all, unnecessary."

Dr. Shafer told a news conference that one aim of the commission's final report was "to reorient the attitudes of Americans toward drug abuse."

"The enemy is not drugs or drug use, but the behavioral conduct of certain types of drug users," he said.

The chairman said that the study had indicated that people did not turn to drug use when "a satisfactory alternative" was available to them. Such alternatives, he said, were, for example, for the poor "a chance to work" or, for middle-class people, "purposeful political or environmental activity." . . .

The report took the position that the Government should not interfere with an individual's decision to use drugs that might be harmful to his personal health as long as they did not lead him to commit antisocial acts.

"When the risk associated with a type of drug dependence does not involve drug-influenced behavior, but is rather limited to possible danger to individual health," the report said, "it is the commission's view that private normative choices should prevail."

The commission called dependence on alcohol "without question the most serious drug problem in this country today," with addicts far outnumbering those associated with any other drug. About 10 percent of drinkers are compulsive, the report said, half of whom show "a serious decrement in social functioning."

Strongly opposed by the Shafer Commission were sweeping proposals for treatment of all drug users, such as all persons detected using marijuana. It called the proposals "over-reactive and misguided."

Reported Experience With Drug Use for
Recreational and Nonmedical Purposes
by American Youth and Adults
Based on 1972 Survey

	Youth (Ages 12-17)		Adults (18 and Over)	
	Per-cent	Population	Per-cent	Population
Alcoholic beverages*	24	5,977,200	53	74,080,220
Tobacco, cigarettes*	17	4,233,850	38	53,114,120
Proprietary sedatives, tranquilizers, stimulants†	6	1,494,300	7	9,784,180
Ethical sedatives†	3	747,150	4	5,590,960
Ethical tranquilizers†	3	747,150	6	8,386,440
Ethical stimulants†	4	996,200	5	6,988,700
Marijuana	14	3,486,700	16	22,363,840
LSD, other hallucinogens	4.8	1,195,440	4.6	6,429,604
Glue, other inhalants	6.4	1,593,920	2.1	2,935,254
Cocaine	1.5	373,575	3.2	4,472,768
Heroin	.6	149,430	1.3	1,817,062

*Within the last 7 days.
†Nonmedical use only.

Source: National Commission on Marijuana and Drug Abuse

"The experimental, recreational or circumstantial user of drugs is generally no more 'sick' than the social drinker," the report said. "It becomes an absurdity to talk of treating such a person."

Assessing the current drug picture in the nation, the commission said:

"The most serious concern in contemporary America should attach to the use of alcohol and heroin. Moderate social concern should attach to the use of amphetamines, barbiturates, hallucinogens, methaqualone and cocaine, the use of which is relatively well controlled.

Nixon Proposals Ignored

"The use of marijuana and the so-called minor tranquilizers appears to require relatively minimum social concern at the present time. Present trends do suggest, however, that the incidence and use of and dependence on barbiturates and cocaine may be increasing and may demand increased social attention."

The report ignored the most recent recommendations of the Nixon Administration when it referred to "the present disenchantment with prosecution and punishment as a means of dealing with the drug problem."

The commission said that no one should substitute for prosecution and punishment "the facile notion that drug dependence is a disease as susceptible to cure as ordinary maladies of the body."

"Drug dependence is often an illness of the spirit," it said.

In its first report, the Shafer Commission called for an end to criminal penalties for possession of marijuana, a move that the Administration rejected. . . . [In its final report] it added that the drug "does not induce physical dependence" or promote "acts of violence" by its users.

However, the report said, recent studies indicate that marijuana is not good for driving "even at dose levels normally consumed in social settings," since it impairs significantly "visual perceptual performance as well as temporally controlled responses."

MARIJUANA: DECRIMINALIZATION OR CONTINUED PROHIBITION [5]

More than 420,000 persons were arrested on marijuana charges last year, and "pot busts" represented two of three

[5] Reprint of "Report FBI Statistics Show 420,000 Pot Arrests in '73," article by William Hines, staff reporter. Chicago *Sun-Times*. p 10. Jl. 22, '74. Reprinted with permission from the Chicago *Sun-Times*.

drug arrests, according to still-unreleased Federal Bureau of Investigation statistics, a marijuana-law-repeal lobbyist said Sunday.

R. Keith Stroup, director of the National Organization for the Reform of Marijuana Laws, said that when the FBI releases its 1973 Uniform Crime Report, it will show an increase in marijuana arrests of 43 percent over 1972.

The 1973 pot-bust figure—420,700 out of 628,900 arrests for all drug-related offenses—is an all-time high, Stroup said.

A spokesman for the FBI here confirmed the accuracy of NORML's figures. He said the 1973 Uniform Crime Report should be released in about a month.

"This amazing increase in arrests for marijuana is ironic at a time when more and more groups, including the National Commission on Marijuana and Drug Abuse and the American Bar Association, are calling for decriminalization," Stroup declared.

"The costs of continued criminal prohibition, in terms of wrecked lives and careers, is staggering. The costs of law-enforcement resources used to make marijuana arrests, resources badly needed in other areas, are estimated at $250 million to $600 million annually."

"Decriminalization" of marijuana, which Stroup's group advocates, is not the same as legalization. NORML proposes that all criminal penalties for the simple possession and use of marijuana be removed, but that laws against trafficking be retained. "Legalization" of the drug—bringing it to equal status with tobacco and alcohol—is not part of NORML's present reform package.

One state—Oregon—has decriminalized marijuana. Stroup said similar measures are under consideration in several states and in Congress. Little chance is given the congressional proposal to remove marijuana from the list of forbidden drugs.

In his statement on 1973 pot arrests, Stroup said California led the country with 95,110. This accounted for one of every four felony arrests in the nation's most populous state.

A four-year series of statistics compiled by NORML on the basis of FBI reports showed that pot violations as a percentage of all drug arrests increased annually from 1970 through 1973 and that the number of arrests each year increased over the prior year at an ever-accelerating rate.

In 1970, marijuana arrests numbered 188,682 and accounted for 45.4 percent of the 415,500 drug arrests that year. In 1973, marijuana arrests numbered 420,700 and accounted for 66.9 percent of the 628,900 arrests for drug violations.

The 1970–73 increase in the number of marijuana arrests was 19 percent, the 1971–72 increase was 29 percent and the 1972–73 increase was 43 percent, NORML's statistics show.

"This latest data should certainly add impetus to the drive to decriminalize the estimated 26 million Americans who occasionally smoke marijuana," Stroup said.

"We should continue to discourage all recreational drug use, including alcohol and tobacco as well as marijuana. But we should stop making criminals out of those who ignore our advice. Giving a criminal arrest record to the user only exacerbates the potential for harm."

GOING TO POT [6]

Through the local United States attorney here, the Department of Justice has made known that the crime of possession of small amounts of marijuana will no longer be prosecuted.

Because this announcement comes as a welcome relief to many who do not like to see young people "busted" for participating in a prevailing custom, nobody takes notice of a remarkable precedent being set.

The executive branch of Government, through its Attor-

[6] Reprint of essay by William Safire, columnist. New York *Times*. p 47. N. 21, '74. © 1974 by The New York Times Company. Reprinted by permission.

ney General, has just arrogated to itself power formerly held by the judicial branch and the legislative branch.

What right does any law enforcement officer have to decide which laws, passed by local or Federal legislatures, shall be labeled null and void? What right do prosecutors have to usurp the function of judges in deciding that the holder of five marijuana cigarettes shall go free and the holder of six shall be prosecuted?

The right, of course, is the discretion placed in the hands of law enforcement officials; in practice, not one of ten crimes of almost any nature is aggressively prosecuted, because courts and jails are already overcrowded.

But this discretion, or latitude, is given to prosecutors on the assumption that they will act discreetly; it is grossly abused when lawmen publicly announce which laws they have decided not to carry out. The Department of Justice is not in business to make new laws or repeal old laws—that is for congressmen and councilmen alone—and the final decision to mete out justice should remain in the hands of judges.

Our off-the-wall US attorney here has gone to the extent of assuring policemen that they will not be prosecuted for failing to carry out the law. What has happened to the concern so recently expressed about the sinister assumption of power by the executive branch? The concern vanishes when the power is usurped for a purpose popular with most liberals.

The decision on the legalization of marijuana is a matter to be faced squarely by elected officials, not fuzzed up by the fuzz. "Decriminalization" is a foolish euphemism for crime without punishment: If we are not prepared to exact a penalty for the commission of an act, then we should stop calling it a crime.

I think marijuana smoking is harmful and should be legalized. Liquor and tobacco are harmful and legal; a libertarian conservative view is that government should get out of the business of telling people how to conduct themselves when their conduct does not harm others.

At least twenty million Americans smoke pot; the grass has roots. Since prohibition has not worked, regulation should be given a chance. The only effective curb on marijuana use will come from the left, not the right; from the force of health faddism and social pressure, not the force of law.

This week, as elected officials permitted appointees to walk off with their power to legislate under the banner of "decriminalization," the Department of Health, Education and Welfare was coming at marijuana use from its vulnerable left side.

A new HEW report warns that habitual use may depress the male sex hormone, possibly leading to birth defects; it also may lower resistance to disease; and in a classic non sequitur, the report adds that intoxication may lessen the ability to concentrate. As with HEW data on cyclamates, the report plays on fears more than facts—pot has not been proven to be a gaseous thalidomide—but fear does more than evidence can to justify God's ways to man.

In a coming, short-lived era of the cannabisinessman, this is what we could expect: the legal importation, growth and sale of marijuana, heavily taxed by each level of government ("soak the young" is the slogan, but prices should be kept high as a work incentive).

Advertising would be regulated; as with liquor, TV and radio would be banned, and as with tobacco, warnings would be required on all print media. Tests would be developed to measure marijuana intoxication, and the crime of driving while stoned would be vigorously prosecuted.

Most important, the social protest connection would be broken. Smoking pot would be viewed not as "our thing," forbidden fruit, but as a combination of booze and butts, harmful to the human body; substitutes would be sought for mind-expansion that are harmless, like exercise, meditation, self-hypnosis or—who knows?—gargling.

Tests will continue; not to determine whether marijuana is addictive, which was yesterday's argument, but to show whether it is harmful. And it is in the very nature of "scientific tests" to show that the ingestion of anything is ultimately harmful.

Tomorrow's young people, already suspicious of smoking tobacco, will read the scary label of the legal packet of grass: "The Surgeon General warns that smoking pot may cause sexual impotence, birth defects and lower resistance to colds."

Wouldn't that be more effective in curbing the use of an artificial escape from reality than the present method of unenforceable law, or the abdication of legislative responsibility to the Department of Justice?

THERE'S GOLD IN THEM THERE PILLS [7]

The scene has become familiar. A new and dangerous pattern of abuse with a legally manufactured drug is belatedly discovered by the Government. Congress threatens to control it. The pharmaceutical houses that are making a bundle from the drug's popularity oppose the bill. The Food and Drug Administration, the regulatory agency of the drug firms but sometimes their protector, goes to Capitol Hill, pleads for more time to study the problem and promises to take appropriate action later. Meanwhile casualties of the drug climb.

We have seen it happen with amphetamines and barbiturates. This time it is methaqualone, a sedative-hypnotic often prescribed for insomnia. Its effects are similar to those of barbiturate and so are its dangers. A few pills make one drunk; higher doses can result in unconsciousness, coma or even death. The few pills that would otherwise have caused

[7] Excerpt from an article by Peter J. Ognibene, contributing editor. *New Republic*. 168:13-15. Ap. 21, '73. Reprinted by permission of *The New Republic*, © 1973 The New Republic, Inc.

a "high" can become a knockout, possibly fatal, dose when taken with liquor.

Drug firms have been building a safe image for methaqualone in their advertising, much of it in medical publications. These ads have led many people to believe the drug is a nonaddictive "downer" when in fact it is every bit as dangerous as barbiturate. Senator Birch Bayh (Democrat, Indiana), chairman of the Senate juvenile delinquency subcommittee calls methaqualone "the Dr. Jekyll and Mr. Hyde drug, seemingly safe while actually deadly." . . .

In a joint statement, Dr. George R. Gay and Darryl S. Inaba of the Haight-Ashbury Free Medical Clinic in San Francisco told Bayh's subcommittee: "In January of 1973 a short survey of patients seen at the Drug Detox [detoxification] Project revealed that 15 percent reported a past moderate to heavy abuse of methaqualone, 20 percent had tried it 'a few times' and 65 percent had never tried it." . . .

The [former] acting commissioner of FDA, Sherwin Gardner, told the Bayh subcommittee: "Prescription data for the leading methaqualone products show an increase from about one half million in 1968 to about 4 million in 1972. In 1972 there were approximately 111 million 300mg. dose equivalents of methaqualone dispensed by prescription in pharmacies and approximately 185 million dosage units distributed by all manufacturers." One of them, Quaalude, is now "the sixth most popular sedative-hypnotic in the United States," said Gay and Inaba, and "in 1972 Quaalude sales alone increased 360 percent." Produced at a cost of less than four cents per 150mg. tablet, methaqualone has fast become a big money-maker.

Bayh requested representatives of the pharmaceutical houses to appear before the subcommittee. Two refused. (More on that later.) Parke-Davis, which makes Parest, sent one of its vice presidents, Leslie M. Lueck, who told the subcommittee that "the company is of the strong opinion that this drug must be controlled under the Controlled Substances Act of 1970." But Parke-Davis is opposed to the

Schedule II classification in the Bayh bill (S1252). "The drugs now on Schedule II are potentially dangerous and addictive at their normal recommended dosage levels," said Lueck. "Such is not the case with methaqualone at recommended dosage levels." The evidence contradicts these assertions.

Although all the drugs on Schedule II are "potentially dangerous," not all are addictive at "normal recommended dosage levels." For example amphetamine is not addictive at the low dosage levels prescribed by physicians; very high, sustained dosage levels are required for addiction to occur. While methaqualone may also not be addictive when taken as directed for insomnia, addiction has been reported by the University of Michigan Hospital at dosage levels as low as 1.2 grams a day or four 300mg. tablets. If amphetamines had been taken only as directed by physicians, there of course would have been no abuse of the drug. It was the *potential* for abuse, high production levels (eight billion amphetamines a year) and the absence of security requirements that led to the drug becoming so popular with housewives as well as "speed freaks." The growing popularity of methaqualone, its rapidly increasing production levels and its great potential for abuse have created a situation nearly identical to that of amphetamine several years ago. If speed belongs under Schedule II of the Controlled Substances Act, so does methaqualone.

The two drug company presidents who refused to appear before the Bayh subcommittee were J. W. Eckman of William H. Rorer, Inc., the maker of Quaalude, and Robert E. Parcell of Arnar-Stone, the maker of Sopor. (The "street names" most often used for methaqualone are quaalude and sopor.) Bayh called their refusal the worst example of noncooperation he had seen in eleven years in the Senate. With the unanimous support of the subcommittee, he issued subpoenas for the two men to appear before the subcommittee. . . . Predictably, Eckman and the Anar-Stone vice president who represented Parcell recommended against Schedule II;

the latter suggested Schedule III: the same set of ineffective controls that made it possible for amphetamine production to boom to eight billion doses a year.

. . . [In November 1972] the Bureau of Narcotics and Dangerous Drugs amassed a persuasive case for putting the nine short-acting barbiturates under Schedule II and sent it to FDA for its concurrence. In February [1973] BNDD recommended methaqualone be put under Schedule II. Apparently prodded by the Bayh subcommittee, FDA on April 5 concurred with BNDD's recommendation. If the Attorney General accepts these recommendations, he can place the drug on Schedule II. Since amphetamine has been under Schedule II, production quotas have been cut 90 percent, and early this month the Government began making what a BNDD spokesman called "the largest recall of controlled substances ever made" and ordered the recall and destruction of all injectable amphetamines and diet pills that contain the drug. Unfortunately it seems to take a drug epidemic and a large number of deaths or injuries before the Government will get tough with the drug manufacturers and use the law to protect the public from legally manufactured drugs that are being abused.

III. SOCIAL AND MEDICAL ASPECTS

EDITORS' INTRODUCTION

The central section of this volume is a collection of articles on the use of drugs, legal and illegal, in contemporary American life.

To begin with, there is a transcript of about half of a local New York CBS news series, *The Television Report: Drugs A to Z,* in which most of the substances considered to be drugs are listed alphabetically and discussed individually. (The one important deletion the editors have made from the report is the segment on alcohol, which has always been and still is the largest single addiction problem; alcoholism is the specific subject of another article in this section.)

There are next three newspaper articles on the subject of the illicit heroin traffic network, from Turkey via Marseilles to the United States, sometimes known as the French Connection, which achieved even wider notoriety from the movie of the same title.

The following selection concerns the use and abuse of alcohol, with the emphasis on youthful addiction. One of the major difficulties alcohol presents is that unlike the illegal drugs, it is legal, accessible, and—except for a few groups—socially acceptable.

The next two articles deal with what has come to be known recently as polydrug abuse. As the name implies, the problem arises from the fact that there are so many drugs available, with such varying effects and functions, that the drug user or experimenter combines different substances, sometimes dangerously.

The last article in this section is by Dr. Andrew Weil; his studies of methods of drug use employed by a number of South American Indian tribes have produced interesting comparisons between the approach toward drugs of tribal Indians and the prevailing approach in the United States and Europe.

A GLOSSARY OF DRUGS [1]

Amphetamines

Amphetamines are fast becoming a troublesome class of drugs in the United States. With and without doctors' prescriptions, millions of persons now take these stimulating drugs for everything from staying awake at night on the road to passing final examinations. And they are also being used simply for drug experience. The people in the drug underground call them "ups" because they raise emotional level. They are also called "bennies" and "dexies," nicknames for Benzedrine and Dexedrine, two trademark forms of amphetamine. Some are commonly called "speed." To take amphetamines is to speed.

Manufacturers turn out 10 billion pills a year, a production bigger than for barbiturates. In small doses, amphetamines are powerful antifatigue and antisleep pills. Students have known for a long time that using amphetamines will enable them to finish a final paper or cram for an examination. They do extend work ability but they do not decrease the mistakes. Truck drivers use them to stay awake on long rides. One survey suggests that more than half the truck drivers in the United States use these pills. Housewives take them mornings to keep going during the dull chores of housework. Doctors give them to overweight people since amphetamines cut appetite. But while the pills can start weight reduction, they cannot keep the person reduced since he must take more and more amphetamines to achieve the same appetite control. Inhaled, amphetamines

[1] Excerpts from *The Television Report: Drugs, A to Z,* by Earl Ubell. WCBS-TV. 51 W. 52d St. New York 10019. '70. Reprinted with permission from WCBS-TV and the author.

relieve nasal congestion. And although amphetamine is a stimulant, it paradoxically calms down certain types of over-active children.

Overall, with amphetamines doctors can reduce nervous fears, fatigue and other depressed mood complaints. With such power it's no wonder that amphetamines, if uncon-trolled by a physician, can lead to psychological dependence. As with cocaine, amphetamine does not produce physical dependence of the same type that heroin does, but it does create a craving, a very powerful craving which is another form of addiction. This craving, along with the stimulating properties of amphetamine, has turned it into one of Amer-ica's most troublesome drugs. And has done so with one of America's most useful drugs.

The drug underground has taken to amphetamines with a vengeance. Some not only pop the pills but they also sniff the stimulant drug and inject it. A powerful form of am-phetamine called methamphetamine or methedrine is usu-ally used for injection. The drug users call this drug "meth," "crystal," and "speed." Amphetamines have created a whole new class of addicts. They are not physically dependent upon the drug as heroin addicts are, but they can take it for weeks. The amphetamines have produced a class of emaciated, frenetic youngsters, since the drug not only kills appetite but creates wild behavior. Injections of meth can produce hallucinations. Unknown forces sweep over the users and give them a feeling of clarity of vision. They talk, and talk, and talk, and talk, wandering aimlessly in the streets. Then comes a "crash," a feeling of despondency and depression. Doctors know about the fatigue and sadness that follow amphetamines, so when they take their own patients off the drug they do so slowly. But the speed freak crashes every day. His days alternate between frenetic vision and utter depression because he takes more of the drug to lift himself up after each crash.

There is another type of amphetamine speeder. He is the successful businessman, musician, actor, the college professor who is expected to have a high rate of production, so he pops amphetamines to keep going. So high is he on these drugs that at night he must take barbiturates to sleep—so he is on a constant cycle of amphetamine and barbiturate.

Nobody knows what the long-term use of amphetamines does to the human mind and body. Some heavy users are plagued with skin disease. Some individuals show the mental signs of suicide, and even homicidal tendencies have been reported. Ultimately stimulation is followed by fatigue and depression. Inside medical channels the drugs are useful, but outside there is a growing feeling that these drugs can be as dangerous as barbiturates or alcohol.

Barbiturates

Barbiturates are downers. These drugs bring you down emotionally, they relax you. And for those who cannot sleep, they produce sleep. Barbiturates resemble alcohol; in large doses they produce the same drowsiness, the same dull memory, the same slurred speech. And like alcohol, barbiturates do produce some addiction.

The people in the drug underground call them blue heaven, yellow jackets, red devils, red birds, because they come in colored capsules or pills. Manufacturers now produce eighty different combinations of various barbiturates. All are artificially made. And each year the factories turn out close to a million pounds of the drug, or about forty pills for every man, woman and child in this country. Doctors prescribe them to produce sleep in the sleepless, to calm the jittery and to prevent convulsions in the epileptic. Barbiturates, perhaps more than any other drugs, have created the ambience of a pill-taking society. Nervous? Take a barb. Can't sleep? Take a goofball. They've been in use since the turn of the century. And in small amounts, prescribed by physicians, a barbiturate can produce tranquility in a nervous patient.

Aside from addiction, barbiturates have other dangers. People who have used them for a long time accidentally

take too many. They simply forget how many they have
already taken. Because the drug dulls memories, they end
up in the hospital, victims of barbiturate poisoning. Sometimes it's hard to tell if the victim intended suicide. In one
five-year period in New York City alone there were 8,500
cases of barbiturate poisoning. And 1,100 of them died. Half
were called suicide.

Then, too, you cannot mix barbiturates and alcohol.
The alcohol makes the goofball more toxic. The combination dulls reflexes and loosens control over muscles and over
perception. So a person who drives an automobile after having taken a barbiturate and alcohol may be driving himself
and others to the morgue.

Nobody knows exactly how many barbiturate addicts
there are in the United States. It must be several hundred
thousand, since one out of four prescriptions written for a
mood-changing drug is for a barbiturate. And then, too, the
illegal market is huge. It represents a vast, unknown amount
of drugs. Illicit barbiturates are manufactured underground,
stolen or imported. Researchers now believe that the process
of addiction to barbiturates is similar to that of addiction
to alcohol, but many doctors say that barbiturate addiction
is even harder to treat than heroin addiction.

The process starts with small amounts of the drug which
produce relaxation and a sense of well-being. Then the patient finds he needs more and more of the drug to get the
same effect. The experts call this building up a tolerance.
Simultaneously, the barbiturate user becomes mentally dependent on the drug. He craves it just as an alcoholic craves
a drink. Finally, if the barbiturate user tries to get off the
pills, he suffers withdrawal sickness: cramps, dizziness, convulsions and sometimes a sudden and painful death. It's the
alcohol addiction pattern all over again, with a different
drug. The fear of withdrawal keeps the barbiturate user
going even though he no longer enjoys the same effects as
he once did.

Most barbiturate-dependent persons are middle-aged,

and the middle-class housewife is well represented among the addicted groups. Although it has not been as intensely studied as alcohol addiction, barbiturate abuse probably has come about in a similar way. We live in a society which approves the taking of pills to relieve tension, to solve the problems of mental anguish. We see pill-taking advertised everywhere. A potential addict enters the drug-taking scene with overt and implied social approval. The rest follows when his pill-taking is not under the control of, or leaves the control of, a physician.

Technically, only a doctor can prescribe barbiturates, and the laws provide up to fifteen years in jail for those who sell the drug illegally. The laws may have slowed the abuse, but with doctors handing out these drugs as freely as they do, they are creating thousands of illegal users and, therefore, the underground market has been hard pressed to keep up with the increasing demand for barbiturates.

Caffeine

For the average American, the day starts out with a cup of coffee, or a cup of tea or cocoa. Although everybody knows it, few stop to realize that these drinks contain a powerful stimulating drug: caffeine. Caffeine acts directly on the brain. It produces a rapid and clear flow of thought and fights fatigue and drowsiness. Caffeine not only allows a better mental effort, it sharpens the senses. Studies show that typists work faster and with fewer errors. But if you have just learned a new skill that requires delicate coordination, caffeine can increase the number of mistakes. All of these effects are brought on by the caffeine contained in two cups of coffee or tea. Both drinks contain the same amount of the drug. A twelve-ounce cola drink contains about half the caffeine in a cup of coffee, and cocoa contains a chemical cousin of caffeine that produces the same effects.

Not everyone reacts to caffeine in the same way: some can drink one cup of coffee and remain sleepless for the night; others can drink a dozen cups a day and feel no effects. As you drink more, you need more to get the same stimulation. Because caffeine constricts blood vessels in the brain, some people come down with pounding headaches. In the long term, little is known about the bad effects of caffeine. There is one peculiar report linking heart attacks with coffee but not with tea.

As for addiction, science is mute. Unquestionably, some are dependent upon the daily drink of caffeine to keep going, and there are others who, when they stop drinking, crave it. In any case, consumption of this mood-changing drug is massive. Almost 3 billion pounds of coffee, 13 million pounds of tea and 800 million pounds of cocoa are consumed in the United States, to say nothing of cola drinks. Once, long ago, tea was illegal in England and smugglers had their hands chopped off for bringing the drug into the country. It was considered devil's brew. Now that caffeine is firmly entrenched in our country's society and into our country's way of life, other drugs are considered devil's food.

Cocaine

Cocaine may be the most addicting drug known. Animals addicted to cocaine will die of starvation if given a choice of being deprived of food or of cocaine. Cocaine comes from the coca leaf, a plant growing high in the Andes Mountains of South America. There, the Indians working in the rarefied atmosphere pluck the leaves and chew on them to fight fatigue because cocaine is the most potent antifatigue chemical known. The pure chemical taken by mouth, sniffed or injected, creates the quickest stimulation to the brain known. The user becomes restless and talkative. He feels immediate enormous physical strength and great intellectual capacity—both of which he overestimates. There is no question that cocaine takers can work harder and longer at both physical and intellectual work while the drug effects last. Medically, cocaine is a local anesthetic—it dulls feeling where it is injected. However, procaine has largely replaced cocaine in medical use.

Sigmund Freud, the Viennese father of psychoanalysis, first developed cocaine as a local anesthetic in the 1880s. He also recognized the stimulating properties of the drug and he thought that it could be an antidote to morphine addiction. With cocaine, Freud successfully weaned a doctor friend away from morphine. But he also turned his friend into the world's first cocaine addict.

As with other drugs, addiction follows repeated use. The Peruvian natives who chew the coca leaves soon give up the habit when they come down from the high altitudes and no longer need the stimulation. The usual physical dependence of heroin does not follow cocaine addiction. When the drug is stopped, the individual does not feel the same withdrawal symptoms as he would with heroin. But if he does stop the drug, the craving for it is excruciating and he soon falls into a deep state of fatigue and mental despondency, so deep in fact as to sometimes cause suicide.

Cocaine has been called the king of illegal drugs. It is also the most expensive, costing about fifty dollars a gram. Cocaine is extracted as a pure chemical from the leaf of the coca plant. . . . Heroin addicts have been known to mix heroin with cocaine to prolong the effects of heroin. But cocaine users prefer the drug for its stimulating properties. They either inject the pure chemical or, mostly, sniff it. And because cocaine has a deleterious effect on the inner linings of the nose, cocaine sniffers can destroy their nostrils. Cocaine users include musicians, writers, businessmen in high office and even college professors. Since the cost is high and the effects are short-lived, requiring the user to purchase large amounts of the drug, only high-income individuals can afford it. It does generate some crime, but not as much as heroin does because there are more heroin addicts than cocaine addicts. At the turn of the century, probably more persons were addicted to cocaine than to heroin or to other opium products. Sherlock Holmes told Dr. Watson that he used cocaine (probably by injection) and while that was fiction, it may have represented the true state of affairs in the late 1800s.

The cocaine trade starts in South America where the coca plant grows. There, in secret laboratories, chemists extract the drug and then ship it to the United States illegally through Miami and New York. The amount of trade is unknown but it must reach into the millions.

The average cocaine user does not get into trouble. Many do, though, because the drug brings on feelings of persecution, what psychiatrists call paranoia, and then the cocaine addict may act against his imagined persecutors. Cocaine is a powerful drug: if the user takes too much of it, it may stop his heart, stop his breathing and kill him.

Heroin

Heroin or, as the addicts call it, *horse, smack* or *scag,* is the hard stuff. To many it's the horror stuff. Hardly a day passes when one of them doesn't end up in the emergency room, a victim of the drug. Heroin is not the most addicting drug; cocaine takes that prize. And yet heroin arouses the most fear. Part of that fear comes from the associated crime of heroin addiction, and part comes from the fact that it has now spread into the middle-class community.

Heroin is the chemical sister of morphine, and morphine is extracted from opium, which in turn comes from the juice of the seed pod of the opium poppy. Ounce for ounce, heroin is up to ten times more powerful than morphine. Doctors shun heroin as a painkiller only because it is illegal. In the body heroin behaves like morphine, and like alcohol and barbiturates, heroin depresses the nervous system. It is a downer. For persons in pain it kills pain; for normal individuals it can first create a sense of fear, of nausea and sometimes vomiting. After a while it brings on drowsiness, clouds thinking and makes the voice husky. It also eventually produces the deepest imaginable sense of well-being, but the effects last only an hour or two. Years of opiate use do not seem to damage the user physically, but in animals with high dosage there does seem to be brain damage. Heroin reduces sexual drive, thus creating marital difficulties for some. And chronic opiate users, even when they have enough money to pay for the drug, do not seem able to maintain a job or normal human relationships. A few do, but most do not.

Users and addicts of heroin swallow it, sniff it, pack it under the skin—they call it *popping*. But the fastest response comes from injecting it into the vein—that's called *mainlining*. Some addicts also feel a sensation in the lower abdomen which they call a *rush*, and some experts say that rush is a sexual feeling.

The social danger from heroin comes from the crime which the addicts commit to get their drug; and the personal danger to the addict comes from the possible overdose, from the dirty needle and from the burglaries he must commit in order to buy his daily dose.

A hundred thousand Americans, mostly men and mostly in their twenties, live chained to heroin. Some say the figure is close to 250,000. But not all users of heroin are addicts, since it takes time to become dependent upon the drug. And dependency brings with it a life dominated by the drug, by crime, by the fear of overdose, by sickness and by a complete personality change. One theory holds that the drug changes the body chemistry so that it continues to require the drug; it produces a craving. Another suggests that heroin addiction, like that to alcohol, is primarily social and psychological. Social pressures come first. Drug users urge other non-drug users to try it. At first they feel nausea, dizziness and fear. Only social pressure could make a one-time user continue to take the drug. One shot does not make an addict.

Because the drug is illegal, heroin reduces the addict to a hounded creature. With the source of drugs unknown, overdose is a danger. Dirty hypodermic needles infect his liver, his blood, his brain. Prostitution, a common way of earning drug money, brings with it venereal disease. Allergic reactions to heroin contaminated with dirt can kill; amoral addicts have been known to feed each other rat poison instead of heroin. In short, the addicts, who are mostly in their twenties, face a death rate like that of seventy-year-old men.

Every drop of heroin in this country is illegal, and there is no medical application for the drug. With an estimated 250,000 users, there is a market for the drug which does about $100 million to $500 million worth of illegal business every single year. And that supply system gives users small doses, tiny doses, at $5 to $10 apiece.

All the heroin in this country is derived from opium which is grown in Turkey and other Near Eastern countries. The processing and smuggling network rivals the bootlegging operations of Prohibition times. By the time heroin passes through some five stages of illegal handling, it contains less than 2 percent heroin. The handlers add milk sugar, which is white, to provide bulk and then quinine to mask the taste. And street dealers charge something like $5 for a product which costs less than a hundredth of a cent wholesale.

True addicts, who crave the drug daily, generate most of the social problems. They number some 60,000 and they need between $300 and $500 a week for their heroin. Few can afford it. Most turn to stealing. Heroin crime, some estimate, costs the public up to a half billion dollars a year in thefts.

Enslaved to the drug, the addict is hounded by the law on one side and by his dependence on criminal suppliers on the other. And the vise is growing tighter as the penalties grow more severe for heroin trade each year. One who sells to minors, for example, can be sentenced to death in some states. And still the traffic flourishes. The law does not seem to deter the street sellers who oftentimes are themselves addicts. So the law is merely another terror for the addict and it keeps him away from medical treatment.

Some have suggested the free distribution of heroin to

addicts as a way to collapse the market. The method has been tried in England, so far without much success in either containing the drug usage or making useful individuals out of the addicts. Psychological treatment has yielded meager results. Methadone, which is itself a narcotic (a synthetic narcotic), has kept a significant number of addicts out of the heroin market. About a third of heroin addicts leave the drug scene as they grow older, provided they survive long enough to do so, and yet heroin remains one of the most fearful of all the drugs.

LSD

LSD is the most powerful drug known for producing visions or, as scientists call them, hallucinations. The drug has become common on American college campuses where the drug users call LSD "acid." Scientists call it lysergic acid diethylamide. Taken by mouth, less than a millionth of an ounce of LSD will produce, in less than an hour, the most vivid visual distortions imaginable. In 1943, the man who first created LSD, a Swiss chemist, reported that he merely sniffed the material he was synthesizing and soon he "fell into a peculiar state similar to drunkenness, characterized by an exaggerated imagination. With my eyes closed, fantastic pictures of extraordinary plasticity and intensive color seemed to surge toward me."

Since then thousands of persons, mainly in their twenties, have taken LSD illegally. They report a sensitivity to vibrations. They talk of flying through space beyond Saturn, of diving to the center of the earth, of zipping off to China. They tell of auras of vibrating energy around living things, around trees, around clouds.

Imagine the impact of LSD at the Woodstock Music Festival where thousands, reportedly, took the drug. Such experiences are called "trips," and when everything goes well, it is a good trip. Some have called the LSD trip a religious experience. However, there are also bad trips. Some psychiatrists describe the mental state produced by LSD as mimicking the symptoms of schizophrenia, which is a severe mental illness. And some users of LSD have fallen into mental breakdowns that have lasted for years. Doctors agree that it is the individual who is already in mental trouble who may be pushed over the brink by LSD. So the individual who takes the drug for a kick may find himself in a total mental blackout and in a mental institution. In truth, such events are rare. But as more and more individuals take LSD, we will find that more and more of them are breaking down.

Doctors are continually amazed by the fact that less than a millionth of an ounce of LSD can turn the human mind into a ball of fireworks. And they are concerned that in a few individuals LSD also produces mental breakdown. Doctors have tried to treat mental illness with LSD, since the drug mimics some of the effects of mental disease. But they have not succeeded. Some doctors say, and their claim is controversial, that LSD sometimes helps alcoholics. Others use LSD to open a patient to psychological treatment, but again, the efficacy of the technique has been doubted. Aside from mental effects, LSD speeds up the heart, dilates the pupils and sometimes produces a fever. It does not kill, even in large doses. But there are reports—quite rare—of persons who have committed suicide after taking the drug.

Recently scientists reported that LSD may affect the heredity of the offspring of the person taking the drug. In some doses, LSD breaks up the chromosomes, the tiny, rod-like objects in human sperm and egg that carry characteristics from parent to child. But other researchers could not detect chromosome breakup in human beings taking LSD. Again, some doctors say that there are abnormal babies among LSD takers; other scientists have challenged the data. The issue is in doubt. It has received so much publicity, however, that many stopped playing with the drug for fear of maiming their future children.

Doctors also disagree about the addicting properties of LSD. There are no withdrawal symptoms, but some LSD users take the drug again and again, a sign of possible psy-

chological dependence. Even though the drug is now . . .
[more than twenty-five] years old, scientists do not know the
whole story. . . .

Marijuana

In the United States, the marijuana plant has many
names. It's called *pot, mary jane* or *weed;* in cigarette form
it's called a *joint,* a *stick* or a *reefer,* but all are the same top
leaves or the dried flowers of the [hemp] plant, known sci-
entifically as *Cannabis sativa,* so marijuana is also known as
cannabis. In the United States this plant is smoked. The
smoker falls into a dreamy "stoned" state. To the observer,
it doesn't look as though much has happened. But the user
often reports an increase in the sharpness of vision. Apparently the appreciation of music is more intense. The sense
of touch seems more exciting. Most of all, time is slightly
distorted. Seconds seem like minutes, and minutes like
hours. Some users feel exalted and talk of inner joy or happiness.

The user says he is "high." Scientists call all these responses hallucinations and they classify marijuana as a mild
hallucinogenic drug. However, the marijuana that is grown
and used in the United States is not so powerful as the non-
user believes. Often, those who try it feel no effect the first
or second time. One theory holds that the body's responses
to marijuana are so minimal that the user must train himself
to recognize them.

The active ingredient of cannabis has been isolated and
synthesized by chemists. It is called tetrahydrocannabinol.
Tests with this drug show no short-term dangerous effects in
animals or in man. There are some reports—and they are
rare—of psychological panic and there are other reports,
even rarer, of real mental breakdown.

As for long-term effects, science is silent. There are some
experts who believe that marijuana is no more dangerous
than coffee or tea, but some say that long-term, continued
marijuana smoking does produce personality changes. All

agree that there are marijuana habitués—potheads—who are
so exclusively concerned with the drug and its use that they
can think of nothing else. However, in a comparison of what
is known of alcohol and marijuana, alcohol proves to be
the more dangerous drug; alcohol is addictive, which marijuana is not; alcohol produces aggressive behavior, which
marijuana does not; alcohol kills and marijuana, as far as
is known, does not.

Marijuana has become the young people's leisure-time
drug and their anger is rising over their feeling that the US
marijuana laws are turning them into criminals. There are
perhaps 10 million youngsters, maybe even 20 million, some
say, who now smoke marijuana regularly. And . . . [in 1970]
a small vocal minority of them gathered in Washington to
flout the law and call for legalization of the drug just as
alcohol is legal.

They want it to be sold just as alcohol is. Those who
want to legalize marijuana say the drug is safe, safer than
alcohol, maybe even safer than ordinary tobacco cigarettes.
They say they have a right to do with their own bodies what
they want to do.

Countering, those who oppose legalization of marijuana
say the drug may have unforeseen long-term dangers. They
point out that it took years to discover the disease-producing
properties of ordinary cigarettes. They also say that because
alcohol is legal and dangerous is no reason to legalize another dangerous drug.

The law severely punishes for possession or selling the
drug. In some states, the sentence is life imprisonment. Mere
possession can mean prison for a college student. Usually,
marijuana smokers, like tobacco users, give or sometimes sell
friends some of the drug. That act, far from a commercial
underground enterprise, can wreck a life. Among marijuana
users there is a growing feeling that, because adults have
their alcohol, the young should be allowed their pot. They
feel the severe laws only permit adults to control the young.

The tide for marijuana legalization is rising. There are

many who believe that marijuana will soon join alcohol, coffee and cigarettes as legal mood-changing agents for those who want and need it.

Marijuana is illegal in this country. There is also a wide-scale campaign to control and to exterminate this plant and its use as a drug. That campaign is costing millions of dollars. There is the nagging feeling that although science has not proved that marijuana is very harmful, there must be something wrong with it.

By now there is wide agreement that pot or marijuana as it is used in this country does not produce criminals or criminal acts—except by sale or possession. There is also agreement among experts that pot rarely generates mental disturbances, and if it does, the disturbance lasts only a short time; at least in the short run, pot, marijuana, the weed . . . call it what you will . . . does not physically harm the user. There are those who claim that marijuana leads to heroin because almost every heroin addict smoked marijuana before he turned to hard drugs. From the smokers' point of view, however, only a tiny fraction of pot users do turn to heroin, and so they say the connection is not proved.

The antimarijuana faction claims that if pot were more freely available, like alcohol, then the users would turn to more concentrated forms of the drug. They would begin to use hash, or hashish, which is also an ingredient of the hemp plant. It would be as if beer drinkers turned to whisky. Then, they say, the bad effects would show up more frequently.

Hash is increasing dramatically in this country. Hash has more of the active ingredient, tetrahydrocannabinol, in more concentrated form. In Eastern countries it is the preferred form, but in this country the hash used is still very weak. Panic reactions have been reported in connection with hashish use, but they do not last long. And some college medical officers report that marijuana and hash users drop out of college more often, with their competitive drives reduced.

Educators now worry about the overkill propaganda

drive against pot. They feel that when young people learn that the horrors painted for them against marijuana are far from the truth, they will also tend to doubt official word on drugs like heroin, amphetamines, and other drugs which are potentially enormously damaging. In the end marijuana is the most troubling drug. It looks safe—at least now it does— but the laws against it may be generating a criminal element among our young people.

Mescaline

The prickly peyote cactus grows in the southwestern United States and in Central America. The top of the cactus, the "button," contains one of the most powerful drugs known to produce visions, or hallucinations. That drug is mescaline. It was isolated in pure form in 1896, and now it has found its way into the American drug underground.

A hundredth of an ounce of mescaline produces the same sort of visions that LSD does. And different people see different things. Some see color drained away from a room. Others see oranges and reds glow. Some users have the impression of floating forward in time or of standing still in time for what paradoxically seems years. A dog or an animal will stand out from its background and take on an aspect of divinity. For many the effect is exalting and many people maintained that mescaline put them in touch with God. For others mescaline can be deeply frightening even though the main effects last only four to ten hours. Some users report "flashback" recurrences at odd moments. As far as has been determined, mescaline does not produce either physical or psychological addiction. For centuries, American Indians have known about the exalting effects of mescaline. And, in fact, the Native American Church, which combines native lore with some parts of Christianity, uses peyote in ritual. Other mescaline users who claim that the religious usage is important to them have repeatedly been denied any license to use this drug.

Some doctors have used mescaline to treat severe mental

illness like schizophernia, but without much success. In some ways, mescaline can mimic the symptoms of schizophrenia and in some persons, make submerged mental imbalance flare up.

Underground dealers sometimes substitute other drugs for mescaline. One study showed that of a number of drugs sold on the street and labeled mescaline, none contained the drug. They all contained, instead, LSD. Nevertheless mescaline is in wide use and especially among the young users of marijuana and LSD.

Morphine

In the Civil War, morphine, as well as gunshot wounds, inflicted thousands of casualties. Soldiers were the first to receive morphine to ease the pain of their wounds; and at about the same time morphine as a drug was distributed widely in patent medicines, without government control. As a result more than a hundred thousand Americans were addicted to the drug before World War I. Contrary to popular belief, narcotics addiction was then largely a white man's burden. It did not become part of ghetto life until after World War II.

Morphine is one of the many constituents of opium, which itself is a mixture of other narcotics extracted from the seed pod of the opium poppy. Opium, for example, also contains codeine, which is a popular ingredient in cough medicine. Opium use goes back before recorded history. It did not become popular in the Orient until the eighteenth century, but it never was abused there as much as alcohol was in Europe at about the same time.

Medically, morphine is used to kill pain and it does that very well. In individuals in pain it also reduces worry and creates a sense of well-being. Used in that way, under a doctor's prescription, it rarely produces addiction. Given to persons not in pain, it at first produces fear, nausea and often vomiting; so it takes repeated use of morphine for one to become addicted, to get that feeling of well-being that the drug produces. Today the drug can be obtained illicitly, and addicts call it "the white stuff." When they stop taking the drug, they usually suffer the withdrawal symptoms—chills and nausea, cramps and jitters.

Ironically, heroin was invented in Germany as a way to cure morphine addiction. Chemists had been searching for decades for nonaddicting painkillers because they knew what morphine could do. They thought they had found one in 1939 in Demerol, which chemically is dissimilar from morphine; but it too produces addiction and, indeed, many doctors, nurses and pharmacists are addicted to Demerol.

In World War I German chemists synthesized another drug, methadone, which they thought was nonaddicting; but that too proved false and many Germans became addicted to it. So the search for a nonaddicting painkiller has proved to be almost in vain.

Nicotine

Americans smoke nearly 2 billion pounds of tobacco a year and they pay nearly $3 billion for it. By any definition that includes marijuana as a drug, tobacco is a drug. So far, scientists have discovered far more dangerous properties in tobacco than they have in marijuana. It may turn out that in the long run, marijuana may have danger in it just as tobacco does, but it took scientists many years to find out that tobacco had bad properties.

The important chemical in tobacco is nicotine. It is one of the most powerful poisons known. The amount of nicotine in pure chemical form found in two cigars would kill an adult. As a mood-changing drug, nicotine is a stimulant. In the brain, nicotine gives the smoker the well-known "lift." It also speeds the heart and breathing. Like amphetamines, nicotine cuts the appetite. When a youngster first tries to smoke, he feels dizzy, nausea and a choking sensation. As with most drugs, the user has to learn to appreciate the stimulating effects of nicotine.

There is a controversy over whether nicotine is addicting.

Among the 50 million smokers of cigarettes in this country certainly 20 percent of them may be addicted to the drug; that is, they may be physically dependent upon it. When they quit, they actually feel physical symptoms—dizziness, chills and shakes. Many more are habituated psychologically. They cannot seem to stop smoking. Perhaps that's why so few low-nicotine cigarettes have been successful. The nicotine is essential for the enjoyment, and the smoker craves the drug.

In the long run, cigarettes may cut life short by inducing lung cancer, heart attack and various lung diseases. Some of these diseases may be caused by substances in the cigarette smoke other than nicotine, in what is commonly called the "tar." Although the tobacco industry denies the connection between these diseases and cigarette smoking, the preponderance of scientific opinion and evidence holds that cigarette smoking is dangerous. Tobacco is a legal drug, government controlled and taxed. While voluntary health organizations now fight smoking, and . . . [TV advertising of cigarettes was banned in 1971], there has been no move to outlaw tobacco.

Tranquilizers

Chemical tranquilizers for mental illness are among the great medical discoveries of the twentieth century. Those drugs have kept mental institutions from being packed with patients. Drugs like chlorpromazine have calmed the frenzy of mania and reduced the bizarre behavior of psychosis. And others like imipramine have pulled the despondent mental patient out of the depths of depression. These are the so-called major tranquilizers and so far they have not been abused. But they have brought with them a great medical movement to treat mild mental illness with pills. These are the illnesses of anxiety, of fear and depression.

And now we have the minor tranquilizers. Almost every medical journal contains advertisements exhorting doctors to prescribe pills to treat minor mental ills. The most commonly prescribed minor tranquilizers are Valium, Miltown and Librium. All reduce anxiety but the manufacturers warn against giving them to persons who seem to latch on to drugs and take more and more of them against doctors' advice. They also say that in prescribed doses none produces either physical or psychological dependence. However, if a person has been taking any of them for a long time and then suddenly withdraws, he will suffer symptoms, even including perhaps convulsions and coma. Many doctors say that these withdrawal symptoms mimic those produced by barbiturates.

Inside medical channels, there seems to be little abuse of Valium, Miltown or Librium. Some doctors have been criticized for handing them out too freely. Careful physicians test the blood of patients taking these drugs for a long time to guard against blood damage.

There have been some reports of abuse of the minor tranquilizers. Some who have legal prescriptions for them hand the pills out to their friends. And others, who have been discontinued by their physicians, seek out the pills from the drug underground because they need the calming influence. There is some worry in official circles that minor tranquilizers may become the same kind of problem that barbiturates are now. But they are not a problem at this moment.

THE POPPIES OF ANATOLIA [2]

A totally unnecessary confrontation is brewing between the United States and Turkey; unless it can be talked out in terms of reason and good will, serious resentment could erupt to jeopardize Western security interests in the eastern Mediterranean.

The issue is the cultivation of poppies for opium, banned by the Turkish government since 1971 after lengthy discussions with the United States. Under nationalistic political pressures at home, the new Turkish government is giving

[2] Reprint of editorial. New York *Times*, p 16. My. 27, '74. © 1974 by The New York Times Company. Reprinted by permission.

serious consideration to lifting the ban. Against such a possibility, demands are being raised in Congress to suspend all
economic aid to Turkey, a drastic move which could weaken
the Turkish commitment to the North Atlantic Treaty
Organization.

Both sides have a grievance in this complex misunderstanding. For American authorities the Turkish ban is central to the increasingly successful campaign against heroin
addiction. United Nations and Federal Government drug
enforcement authorities point to a dramatic decrease in the
amount of illicit heroin reaching the streets of New York
and other eastern seaboard cities; an estimated 80 percent
of heroin formerly came from Turkey through the illicit
"French Connection" network. Though there are other potential sources of raw opium—particularly Southeast Asia—
international efforts there have scored notable success in dis-
rupting new illicit channels of supply.

From the Turkish point of view, however, the ban has
been a deprivation for some, for others a provocation. Poppies are a traditional and legitimate crop for a small but real
segment of Turkey's farm population—not for opium but
for the edible oil, seeds and stalks. The $36 million Ameri-
can aid program to compensate Turkish farmers for lost
income has, by all accounts, failed—little of the money ever
reaching the farmers themselves. Turkish anger has been
aroused by misleading reports that the United States is encouraging opium production elsewhere, for pharmaceutical
needs. Fortunately an official plan to cultivate poppies in
this country for that purpose has been definitively shelved.
Some Turkish politicians have turned the ban into an emotional issue of national pride.

The way out of this apparent impasse lies not through
threats and acts of national defiance by either side. If the
American aid program has been ineffective so far, it should
be revised and strengthened—not necessarily with more
money, but by better implementation, including small-scale
industrial projects to convince the Anatolian farmers, and

their mentors among the politicians, that they have something to gain by abandoning their poppy crop.

The Turkish government has already shown readiness to remove one irritant to Turkish-American relations; an amnesty measure has reduced the life sentences passed on several young Americans arrested in possession of drugs, though the remaining prison sentences may still seem excessive to many in this country. With a modicum of good will, and recognition of each other's legitimate concerns, there is no reason why both sides cannot benefit from continuation of the Turkish poppy ban. [As noted in the two selections that follow, Turkey rescinded the poppy ban in 1974. Turkish-American relations were further strained by the controversy over continued military aid to Turkey after the Turkish invasion of Cyprus in July.—Eds.]

NEW SURGE IN HEROIN SUPPLY [3]

Special [New York City] narcotics prosecutor Frank Rogers . . . called the Turkish government's decision to resume wide-scale opium production "devastating."

And the head of the [New York City] Police Department's narcotics bureau predicted the move would rapidly create a new influx of heroin. . . .

The two top narcotics officials said that, since the Turkish opium ban was imposed in 1972, law enforcement agencies have been able to reduce significantly the heroin supply here by concentrating their efforts on Asian drug networks.

The European network, sometimes called the "French Connection," was considered to have resources vastly superior to other illicit drug channels and was said to be responsible for 80 percent of all heroin reaching US shores before the ban.

"To me, we're back in the soup again. I can't think of

[3] From "Fear Surge in Heroin Supply Here," article by Jack Cowley, staff reporter. New York *Post*. p 1+. Jl. 3, '74. Reprinted by permission of New York *Post*, © 1974, New York Post Corporation.

anything more devastating," said Rogers. "We were making significant inroads."

Deputy Chief Daniel Courtenay, commander of the police narcotics division, speculated that it would cost the Government four or five times the amount spent on foreign aid to Turkey even to attempt to check the new drug inflow.

The United States granted $35.7 million to the Turkish government under the 1972 pact to compensate farmers for the ban.

"It's an area we felt we had closed down," Courtenay said. "Some addicts have turned to the 'polydrug culture,' methadone, cocaine and others, but now the problems that will be created could be unlimited."

In lifting the ban this week, the Turkish government said that it would allow poppy cultivation to resume in six provinces and part of a seventh.

Opium has medicinal uses, and is the base for morphine, but it has never been determined how much of Turkey's opium production has been sold for medical use.

Police Commissioner Michael Codd said that any such overproduction "in excess" of world market needs can only exacerbate "the conditions and situations with the result being that the excess will go to the underworld."

THE OPIUM OF THE PEOPLE [4]

The opium of the people in Turkey is not religion but politics or, put another way, opium is the politics of the people in terms of an agitated argument with the United States that is not adequately understood by either side.

Premier Bulent Ecevit assured me that "the Turkish government is not emotional on this but in the areas where it is grown, the entire peasant economy depends on the poppy. Therefore the curb imposed in 1971 stirred up psycho-

[4] Reprint of article by C. L. Sulzberger, author and columnist. New York *Times.* p 25. Ag. 24, '74. © 1974 by The New York Times Company. Reprinted by permission.

logical reaction. Opium areas have been reduced by natural
process from forty-two to seven provinces and will be reduced further as new livelihoods appear. We will do what we
can to control illegal traffic but world medicine needs more,
not less, opium."

Poppy growers depend not only on the sap from which
the drug derives but also on flour, fuel and oil extracted
from the plant. And the Anatolian peasant is sometimes at
the lowest subsistence level. Professor Ragip Uner, an expert, says: "In Turkey there are still people who live in
caves and burn oil lamps."

The United States pledged . . . [$35.7] million three years
ago when a ban was announced by Turkey in accord with
Washington. Nevertheless, the government of Konya Prov-
ince, which now resumes cultivation on a small scale, says the
money was slow in reaching actual growers. Substitute crops
weren't swiftly introduced and peasants found themselves
idle. This became a psychological problem.

The Turks make surprisingly little out of opium. Between 1967 and 1971 the annual crop ranged between 120
and 350 metric tons. (It takes ten metric tons of opium to
make one metric ton of heroin.) The grower . . . was getting
perhaps $75 a kilogram for raw opium gum and now might
receive roughly $200. But the retail price of heroin,
smuggled out of this country, processed, then sold in New
York, is about $400,000 a kilogram.

It isn't the farmer who got the vast differential, but the
crook. The moonshining peasant holds back a minor share
of his crop from the government purchasing agency, sells it
to a local bootlegger who sneaks it along to refiners and
transporters elsewhere. Although . . . [Turkey] grows far
fewer poppies than India, it is said 80 percent of US heroin
derives from Turkish gum.

On June 30, 1971, Premier Nihat Erim (whose government was put in by the military) prohibited opium production. He said: "Illicit traffic from our country has become
very distressing"; Turkey had been "unable to prevent smug-

gling"; and "we cannot allow Turkey's supreme interests
and the prestige of our nation to be further shaken."

But politics got into the question as full democracy returned. The minority Ecevit government is based on a coali-
tion. The vote of the poppy growers was needed and all
parties courted it. Were an election to be held now, in the
wake of the Cyprus landing, Mr. Ecevit would win by a
landslide. [Ecevit took office in January 1974 and resigned
in September.—Eds.] But the ban was rescinded July 1, just
before Cyprus exploded.

Politicians argued that farmers were being oppressed,
that there was a world shortage of medicinal opium, that the
United States was turning to India as a source, that anyway
America had no right to boss Turkey. Professor Uner writes:
"No other country has any right to dictate what we have to
cultivate or not to cultivate." But he acknowledges that
Turkish opinion doesn't realize the "hysteria" in the United
States prompted by drug addiction.

American politics is also involved. The United States
Congress, influenced by exaggerated statistics, felt its own
Government wasn't doing enough. To propitiate Congress,
American Ambassador . . . [William B. Macomber, Jr.] was
withdrawn from Ankara right after the restoration of poppy-
farming. Mr. Macomber had to fly back out of the opium
frying pan into the Cyprus fire.

There has been inadequate understanding on both sides.
Americans cannot grasp the misery of impoverished poppy
farmers—or the significance of their vote. The Turks cannot
even imagine the horrors of mass addiction among American
youth. It is certainly imperative that smuggling . . . (which
Mr. Erim admitted was "impossible to prevent") be curbed
and that the criminal chain from farmer to addict be broken.

But it would be well for both nations to remember the
tolerance of Mevlana, a thirteenth century philosopher-poet
who founded the whirling dervish order . . . and counseled
the fanatical medieval world: "Our center is not one of
despair. Even if you have violated your vows a hundred

times, come again." The word "try" should be substituted
for "come."

ALCOHOLISM: STILL THE PRIME
DRUG PROBLEM [5]

A teenager blacked out and fell to the hallway floor of a
Queens [New York City] high school. Unconscious, he was
examined by school officials who concluded that his condition was due to heavy drinking.

We have bad news, a counselor told the boy's mother
over the phone, Johnny passed out at school today. Is it
drugs?, the mother asked. No, it was liquor, the school aide
replied.

"Thank God," the mother said.

The American people over the years have had an am-
bivalent, almost widely cyclical attitude toward alcohol.
Crusades against the Demon Rum have been followed by
periods of unconcern or apathy. Concentrated efforts to find
cures, and sympathy, for alcoholism's victims have alternated
with periods of permissiveness or treatment of drunks as
sodden wrecks, criminals, or clowns.

In recent years, as the story of the Queens student suggests, mounting public panic over drug addiction not only
downgraded alcoholism as a national concern, it almost
made excessive drinking seem frivolously trivial.

And the vocabulary of these addictions, liquor and drugs,
reflected this emphasis. Liquor is respectable; heroin is not.
Drunk is funny; overdose is tragic. Hangover inspires amusement or sympathy; withdrawal terrifies. And so it goes—bar-
tender versus pusher, tavern versus opium den.

Yet, as national statistics indicate, alcoholism has remained unchallenged as the No. 1 addiction problem in
this country, both before and during the relatively recent

[5] Reprint of "Still Problem No. 1," article by Andrew Soltis, staff reporter.
New York *Post*. p 25. Je. 22, '74. Reprinted by permission of New York *Post*,
© 1974, New York Post Corporation.

surge of drug use. And now, as the public outcry over drug addiction seems in recent months to have subsided, we appear again to be redirecting national attention to alcoholism—with special emphasis on the mounting numbers of youthful drinkers. Some authorities, citing the 450,000 American teenagers with a "drinking problem," say that it is none too soon.

. . . [In June 1974 Governor Malcolm] Wilson signed new legislation which by 1976 will "decriminalize" public intoxication and recognize legally what doctors have been saying for years—that alcoholism is a disease, not a moral failing. . . . [Earlier in 1974], the nation's first hospital program directed at treating youthful alcoholics opened at Columbus Hospital [in New York City] under city financing. And a new body, the Advisory Council on Youthful Alcohol and Drug Abuse, was set up this year by the [New York City] Department of Mental Health and Mental Retardation Services to explore initiatives of aid for the reported 66,000 teenage alcoholics in the city.

Alcoholism is clearly a costly disease. Half of the [New York City] metropolitan area's violent deaths, including suicides, accidents and homicides are associated with alcohol, according to the Medical Examiner's office. In recent years as many as one fifth of the New Yorkers who died of drug addiction were also alcoholics and half of all narcotic deaths had alcohol in their body tissues at the time of autopsy.

Alcoholism costs the city millions of dollars annually in industrial losses from absences and inefficiency. The National Council on Alcoholism has estimated there are 2.6 million untreated alcoholics at work in American businesses. The city began its own program . . . [in 1972] for treating municipal workers at detoxification centers.

Drinking and alcoholism, of course, are not the same thing. The Gallup Poll earlier this month [June 1974] concluded that 68 percent of the country's adults (eighteen years and older)—or 95 million people—occasionally use

alcoholic beverages. This marks a 4 percent hike over
the last poll taken in 1969. Furthermore, Gallup reported
that his sampling showed nearly one out of every four persons conceded he sometimes drinks too much. Going one
step further, it was found that one person in eight said
liquor was a source of trouble in his family.

Doctors, psychiatrists and therapists—the people who
treat alcoholism—tend to use a narrower definition of an
alcoholic—"a person who cannot control his drinking
habit." He may want to stop but for medical, chemical or
psychological reasons that have never been adequately answered, he can't. Slightly different is "a drinking problem,"
which could mean a heavy drinking habit just barely under
control. There are perhaps 9 million alcoholics or problem
drinkers in the country.

But youthful drinkers—many of whom were excluded in
terms of age by the Gallup Poll—are a much more complex
problem. "Kids drink for much the same reasons that they
take drugs," John Guerin, director of the [New York City]
Bureau of Alcoholism Services, said. And these reasons are
not the same as those of the middle-aged adult drinker.

"Teenagers have several different kinds of pressures that
adults have forgotten," said Leona Lovell, director of psychiatric social workers of the ACCEPT alcoholism treatment
program at Columbus Hospital. "For example, academic
pressures are not at all like business pressures. There is also
parental pressure and sexual problems. This a time for
young people when they are evaluating themselves and may
be quick to label themselves failures."

There are other complications. To be treated by an anti-
alcoholism program, a teenager needs parental consent.
"But a large number of alcoholic youths come from alcoholic families and the alcoholic parent doesn't want his own
problem exposed through his child's treatment," said Joel
A. Bennett, executive director of ACCEPT.

Also, "There is a growing 'polydrug' problem," said
Arthur Jaffe, of the [New York City] Board of Education's

SPARK program which handles both drug addiction and alcoholism through counseling in the ninety-six public high schools. "Kids are taking 'downers' and booze at the same time and that is very dangerous."

The pattern of youthful alcoholism tends to support the belief that there is an addictive or compulsive personality type which could result in drug addiction or alcoholism or compulsive gambling, or overeating, etc. "We're dealing with a lot of kids who used drugs before and then became scared when the new drug law [in New York State] went into effect in September [1973]. Now they're drinking," said AC-CEPT's Miss Lovell.

Teenage alcoholism is relatively such a new subject of concern that nobody really knows whether kids will be easier to treat than adults.

The majority of alcoholics follow this pattern during their drinking career [said Bennett, who is also cochairman of the city's new Advisory Council]. For a long period of time they continue to function normally without a significant drop in the work performance or their relations with other people. It's only after a long period that they suddenly drop off and can't handle the situation any more.

Now, there is a second category of alcoholics who start drinking and almost immediately begin to have problems. They continue to go down steadily until someone intervenes. For these people it's much more difficult to get them back to the level of functioning normally. And that is where most teenage alcoholics are. They've only been drinking for a year or so before they have trouble. . . .

The National Council of Alcoholism last year [1973] reported that the youngest alcoholics coming to them for help were twelve years old; previously, the group said, the youngest were fourteen.

But the picture isn't completely bleak. "Teenagers haven't acquired the hangups of older people towards the stigma of alcoholism. Adults are hurt by a conspiracy of society which condones drinking and condemns the victim,"

Bennett said. "But kids may be more willing to seek treatment and admit they have a problem."

Treatment comes in a variety of ways. ACCEPT has a twenty-bed in-patient unit, an out-patient clinic with forty weekly therapy groups for all ages and a new twenty-three-bed Halfway House. In addition to medical treatment when necessary, the group offers individual and group therapy, vocational counseling and, in some cases, family counseling.

The nation's oldest and largest anti-alcoholism organization is Alcoholics Anonymous, with 650,000 members worldwide. AA relies on recovery through personal ties with other current and former alcoholics who talk members out of relapsing into drinking. The organization also has allied units, Al-Anon and Alateen, for relieving the problems of the spouses and children of alcoholics.

Treatment of teenagers, however, is likely to be more complex than treatment of adults, Bennett said. And even adult treatment is just scratching the surface.

"In the city there are some 300 hospital beds and through 12 funded programs we can handle an in-patient and out-patient population of about 30,000," Bennett said. "The estimate of the total number of alcoholics in the city—and that is a ten-year-old estimate—is 300,000."

We are apt to think of alcoholics as pathetic, old, skid-row men with weak wills and little natural intelligence or ability. The stereotype doesn't fit even 5 percent of the alcoholic population. The out-patient census of the ACCEPT adult program, for example, shows that most people under treatment are employed, more than a third are married and a third are women. The Gallup Poll sampling showed that among the people who concede they sometimes drink more than they should, the largest category were those who earn more than $25,000, have gone to college and are under thirty years old.

Although alcoholism has been recognized as a health danger and social menace for centuries, there is surprisingly little known about the problem. About $350 million is being channeled into research by the Federal Government over the next two years to answer such basic questions as: what are the effects of liquor on the body; what makes a person vulnerable to alcoholism; what's the best method of treatment?

Alcohol is a strange drug. The stomach manufactures it in small amounts. Alcohol was once frequently kept in medicine chests as a cure-all. It can be useful even today in bedridden patients intravenously because it does not waterlog the body or endanger blood vessels the way that other high-calorie solutions do. A shot of liquor may variously act like a stimulant, a depressant, an analgesic, a sedative or an anesthetic.

The exact relationship between drinking and disease is uncharted. Just recently, doctors reported that one traditional belief—that cirrhosis of the liver is caused by malnutrition rather than alcohol intake—has been refuted. It was further reported that the alcohol itself—rather than impurities added for color or taste—was the greatest danger to the liver. On the other hand, at the American Heart Association's annual meeting . . . [in 1973] it was suggested that a study of the records of the nation's largest prepaid medical plan indicates that social drinkers had fewer heart attacks than teetotalers.

In the past thirty years there has been considerable effort to find the magic chemical which will give the alcoholic back his control over drinking. The first significant discovery came in 1947 when two Danish chemists, Erik Jacobsen and Jens Hald, accidentally found that a compound called disulfiram, which they had hoped could be used to kill intestinal parasites, caused people to become violently ill after drinking cocktails.

The result of this serendipity goes by the trade name of Antabuse and flourished in the early 1950s as the "magic cure." Taken daily in tablets of 500 miligrams at the start of treatment, it was found that Antabuse had no physical effect except when it came in contact with alcohol in the body. However, many doctors turned against the chemical when it was reported that several patients had died after insisting on drinking while under Antabuse medication.

Many psychiatrists who worked with alcoholics also complained that (1) some patients, especially men, refused to take Antabuse because it was "a crutch" and, (2) Antabuse could only be effective if the patient is conditioned by the chemical to adopt a new attitude towards drinking. Today several programs, including ACCEPT, use Antabuse as part of an overall treatment plan that includes therapy and counseling.

Meanwhile, several other chemicals which paralyze the body briefly or cause vomiting when in contact with alcohol have been tried. Few have received any medical acclaim. Recent studies, however, have shown that lithium salts, used since the mid-1950s to combat manic-depressive behavior, may be another way of combating the problem. Rather than interacting with alcohol, the salts attack the depression which may lead a person to the bottle.

Similarly, a drug called propanolol, used in some cases for several years to treat angina pectoris, has been suggested as a means of blocking the mood changes brought about by alcohol. The reasoning goes this way: People drink to change their mood. Propanolol counters the mood-changing effect of alcohol. The drinker then finds that alcohol has no effect on his mood and is conditioned to stop drinking.

But there is always the possibility that social and psychological factors are not the only causes.

The preponderance of the evidence currently available [says the Consumers Union report *Licit and Illicit Drugs*] favors the view that the difference [between alcoholics and nonalcoholics] lies in the childhood . . . the social environment and the stresses to which they are exposed as adults. But . . . most researchers through the decades have been *looking* for psychological and sociological evidence. . . . If as much research, energy and ingenuity were devoted to the search for biochemical factors, the preponderance of evidence might soon shift to the biochemical explanation.

POLYDRUG ABUSE [6]

Across the United States, the spread of heroin addiction appears to have slowed significantly. Indeed, in some places heroin use seems to have leveled off or even dropped.

But interviews in a dozen major cities also show that the easing of heroin addiction has not been accompanied by a general decline in the use and abuse of mind-altering drugs.

Allowing for variations of region, age and class, cocaine, methadone and alcohol, and a variety of barbiturates and other "downers"—most notably a sedative-hypnotic known as methaqualone—appear to be increasingly popular street drugs.

And, while it is difficult to gauge the extent of the phenomenon, a considerable number of people appear to be casually using and abusing several drugs in often dangerous combinations—methaqualone and alcohol, or methadone and cocaine.

"Pill popping has become as common as gum chewing when I was in school," asserts a Boston high school teacher.

In San Francisco, a narcotics police officer reports: "Three years ago it was common to have five or six young people collapse in school every day from an overdose of barbiturates. We don't get that any more; the kids are becoming more sophisticated about drugs."

As for heroin, a Chicago drug counselor observes: "Word has gone out to the black community that smack is part of their oppression, and they are sticking to grass and psychedelics and pills, 'uppers' and 'downers,' for their highs."

Polydrug abuse, as the drug-mixing phenomenon is known, appears to be a characteristic of both school-age dabblers and old-time junkies, who are finding it almost impossible to "cop" (buy) good-quality heroin.

[6] From "Mixing of Mind-Altering Drugs Rises as Spread of Heroin Addiction Slows," article by James M. Markham, staff reporter specializing in drug topics. New York *Times*. p 68. Mr. 25, '73. © 1973 by The New York Times Company. Reprinted by permission.

Decline in Deaths

In New York and other large cities, as a result, a "pure" heroin-reaction death is becoming a rarity; dead addicts now usually have several drugs "on board," in the coroners' phrase.

Around the country, direct narcotics deaths, which had been rising steeply, have begun to level out or even drop. A national sample of twenty-five major geographical areas taken by the White House's Special Action Office for Drug Abuse Prevention recorded a 6 percent decline in such deaths—from 1,859 to 1,740—between 1971 and 1972. . . .

"Caution suggests that we should not say that it's over," observed Dr. Jerome H. Jaffe, director of the special action office.

But he says that systematic interviews with addicts in 214 programs around the country tentatively indicated that heroin addiction had peaked in 1969 and has been leveling off since then.

"We're not trying to claim credit for massive changes in drug use," Dr. Jaffe said. But he and others pointed to the following factors that may have contributed to the slow-down in heroin use:

Treatment Efforts

A rapid build-up in treatment efforts, which have, if nothing else, taken thousands of addicts out of circulation and at the same time fostered the idea that junkies are "sick," not "cool."

Federal spending on treatment has rocketed from $28 million in 1969 to $386 million in 1973. There are now 94,000 addicts enrolled in methadone programs (21,000 of them in detoxification and other nonmaintenance facets) and another 70,000 in a host of drug-free programs.

Deterioration in Quality

A steady deterioration in the quality of heroin on the street, compounded by a prolonged shortage that has only begun to ease. The shortage is a result of a stepped-up enforcement campaign, which may in itself have discouraged marginal users from becoming addicts.

Methadone

The spread of methadone as a street drug. Many junkies now use methadone, which is of reliable purity and cheaper than heroin, as an integral element of their habits.

Change in Drug Fashion

In heavily addicted black and Hispanic communities, a change in drug fashion. The decline of the big-time pusher as a "role model" for young people has been hastened by political attacks contending that the "white power structure" has foisted heroin on minority groups to keep them quiet and submissive.

In New York, Detroit and Miami there have been reports of sporadic vigilante campaigns against pushers. Young blacks now often dabble with methadone, alcohol and LSD, which used to be a white middle-class drug.

Esoteric Drugs

Quirky and esoteric drugs crop up in different corners of the nation—Jimson weed in California or an animal tranquilizer known as "Angeldust" in Chicago, Los Angeles and New York—and cocaine use appears to be spreading, largely because of a plentiful supply.

But, across the nation, barbiturates, and especially methaqualone, appear to be in the highest fashion.

"We're winning in reference to heroin," commented Dr. Matthew P. Dumont, director of the Massachusetts Division of Drug Rehabilitation. "However, I'm terrified about the widespread use of barbiturates."

Inappropriately known in some quarters as "soft" drugs —to distinguish them from "hard" drugs like heroin—barbiturates are in fact addictive and, in several ways, much more dangerous than opiates.

While withdrawal from heroin has rarely killed anyone, barbiturate withdrawal, not to mention overdose, can be fatal. Acute barbiturate intoxication accounts for a quarter of all patients admitted to American hospitals for poisoning and the rate is rising, according to a Senate investigation.

Annually, more than three thousand people die of barbiturate poisoning and, while many of these are suicides, it appears that the number of accidental overdose deaths is growing.

Methaqualone

The use and abuse of methaqualone, which in the United States is sold under the trade names Quaalude, Optimil, Sopor, Parest and Somnafac, began about . . . [1971] in the West and Middle West and then spread to the rest of the country.

Developed in India in the early 1950s methaqualone has had a long and disastrous history of abuse in Britain, Germany, Norway, Japan, Australia and elsewhere. It began to be used medically in this country in 1965 and was—incorrectly—hailed as a nonaddictive hypnotic.

"It was one of those things we could see coming, like a train down the tracks, but we did nothing about it," observed Dr. Emil F. Pascarelli, a drug expert at Roosevelt Hospital in New York.

Production of methaqualone, a prescription drug, soared from almost nothing in the late 1960s to 150 million dosage units . . . [in 1972], according to the Bureau of Narcotics and Dangerous Drugs. . . .

To several observers of the drug scene, the production figures for methaqualone furnish another example of the correlation between the availability of a given drug and the extent of its abuse.

The narcotics bureau, which lists methaqualone among the ten most abused substances in the nation, has urged the Food and Drug Administration to put the drug under tighter restrictions similar to those for morphine, codeine and methadone. The National Commission on Marijuana and Drug Abuse [has] echoed this appeal. . . .

Dr. Pascarelli, who has written on the "quiet epidemic" of methaqualone abuse in the United States, says most of the people he has treated for overdose have been young, white and middle-class, with a scattering of Vietnam veterans mixed in.

PEP PILLS AND OTHER DRUGS [7]

A study conducted for the state Health Department suggests that nearly one third of New Jersey's regular users of pep pills are under the age of eighteen.

The study says virtually every student user of amphetamine takes the drug at school. An analysis of the statistics seems to show that 5,000 of the estimated 9,500 regular users in the 14–17 age group may be unemployed male dropouts from school.

At the same time, the study reveals that nearly 2,500 New Jerseyans in the 14–17 age group are regular users of amphetamines and barbiturates.

Although the number of regular marijuana and hashish users in this age group is more than twice as great (56,000) the authors emphasize that barbiturates and amphetamines account for more drug-related deaths and other health crises than any other drug, including heroin. No regular users of heroin were found in the 14–17 age group.

The study, said to be the most exhaustive of its kind ever undertaken in New Jersey, estimates that 60,000 to 80,000 of the 273,000 regular users of amphetamines and barbiturates could be classified as drug users.

The number of regular users of barbiturates was estimated at 127,000, and the number of regular users of diet

[7] From "Pep-Pill Users: 1 of 3 Under 18," article by Earl Josephson, Trenton Bureau staff reporter. *The Record* (Hackensack, N.J.). p A-1+. Ja. 28, '74. Reprinted by permission.

pill amphetamines at 116,000, compared to 200,000 regular users of marijuana and hashish.

The authors define a regular user as one who takes a drug daily, either at present or within the previous six months.

One indicator of abuse, according to the study, is whether a prescription drug is obtained without a prescription or not used as prescribed.

Fifty to 60 percent of the 29,500 regular users of pep pills, generally Benzedrine and Dexedrine, obtained the pills without a prescription or didn't use them as prescribed—a much higher ratio than for diet pills and barbiturates.

Nearly one fourth of the regular pep-pill users were males in the 14–17 age group, and another 7.5 percent were females. Fewer than 9 percent were black, which is significantly less than the black portion of the population.

Unemployed women over the age of 50 represent the most dominant categories of regular barbiturate and amphetamine users uncovered in the study. The authors say this points to the middle-aged and probably middle-class housewife as a major regular user.

This is significant, the authors say, because the presence and misuse of drugs in a household create an atmosphere and accessibility for adolescent experimenters that may have a deleterious impact in future years. . . .

Top Problem

RPC [the survey-conducting Resource Planning Corporation of Washington] listed heroin as the No. 1 New Jersey drug problem because it accounts for the highest proportion of adult drug arrests, although it is second to amphetamines and barbiturates in the number of related deaths and health crises.

The degree of cocaine use was among the most surprising findings to department officials. The survey said there are 17,600 regular users, including the largest proportion in the low income group for many of the drugs (55 percent).

Nearly one in every four is a woman over the age of 50, and one in three is a male in the 18-24 age group. Six percent are under the age of 18.

Of the 200,000 regular users of marijuana and hashish, 81 percent are under 25. College and high school students account for 44 percent, and three of every ten use marijuana and hashish at school. Two thirds of the users are male and more than one in four is classified as upper or upper-middle income.

The report says that marijuana is involved in 48 percent of all the juvenile court cases.

RPC ranks as New Jersey's third most serious drug problem what it calls the emerging pattern of multiple drug use. The authors say this increases the potential for overdose and poses problems for a treatment system geared predominantly to treating abuses of opiate-derivatives.

Three fifths of the heroin users regularly take marijuana or hashish, the report says, while 68 percent of the cocaine users take at least one other drug, frequently a barbiturate or amphetamine. Only 2 percent of the regular marijuana users also take heroin, the report says.

CLUES FROM THE AMAZON [8]

There exist in the Amazonian regions societies that make liberal use of drugs to alter awareness but do not appear to have problems with them. The tastes of these tribes run to stimulants and, especially, halucinogens rather than to sedative-hypnotics or narcotics, and they have available to them a jungleful of potential intoxicants. . . .

The far greater prevalence of hallucinogenic plants in the New World than in the Old—a mystifying difference from the point of view of botany—can be explained by the present theory of consciousness. . . . What is most relevant

[8] From *The Natural Mind*, by Andrew Weil, M.D., writer and researcher on drugs and related questions of altered consciousness. Houghton. '72. p 99-110. Copyright © 1972 by Andrew Weil. Reprinted by permission of the publisher Houghton Mifflin Company.

about all these plants is that they are natural sources of some of the very drugs that are associated with problems in our society. For example, in the summer of 1967, a scientific expedition to the Rio Negro in northwesternmost Brazil observed the use of an intoxicating snuff called *epená* by a tribe of Waiká Indians in the tiny jungle village of Maturacá. Schultes [Richard Evans Schultes, director of the Harvard Botanical Museum], who participated in the expedition, and [Bo] Holmstedt, a Swedish toxicologist, wrote of the tribe:

The Maturacá Waiká store *epená* in a large bamboo tube hanging from the house beams, and it is employed by any adult male singly or in groups at any time as well as during festivals. The tube is kept full, and the snuff, consequently, is always available for use. Every now and then, an Indian will take the snuff, become intoxicated, dance and sing, all alone with the rest of the village going about its usual chores and not paying any heed to him.

The principal ingredient of this snuff is the blood-red resin of a tree of the nutmeg family. In 1969, a group of Swedish chemists, including Holmstedt, reported that the resin contains large amounts of DMT and related hallucinogens. DMT (dimethyltryptamine) has been available in synthetic form on the American black market. It is snuffed, smoked (usually by mixing the crystals with tobacco, marijuana, or mint leaves), or (rarely) injected and is very similar to LSD in its pharmacological effects except that its duration of action is less than thirty minutes (compared to ten or twelve hours for LSD). Because it is so short-acting, the American drug subculture has nicknamed it the "businessman's high."

When I say that Amazonian Indians have no problems with drugs like DMT, I mean that people in these societies do not take these drugs to rebel against parents or teachers, to drop out of the social process, or to hurt themselves. Neither is their drug use in any way linked with antisocial patterns of behavior. And since the drugs, in many cases, are the same ones tied to antisocial patterns of use in the United States, the differences cannot have much basis in pharmacology. What, then, are these Indians doing differently that enables them to live with drugs and not suffer the negative manifestations of drug use?

Conventional scholarship does not help us answer this question because it has never asked it. Although the drug use of South American Indians has been looked at by anthropologists, botanists, and pharmacologists, it has never been studied by anyone interested primarily in alteration of consciousness. Nor has anyone visited these tribes with the express purpose of finding out why they fare better than we do in their relationships with substances that trigger altered states of consciousness.

From my own studies, readings, and observations, I have come to feel that the success of Indian tribes in this regard has to do with the ways they think about drugs and states of consciousness and with certain principles of drug use they have discovered. Above all, they admit to themselves that their world contains many substances with the potential to trigger altered states of consciousness. They do not try to eradicate these substances or prevent people from having access to them. This attitude strikes me as highly realistic in view of the abundance of hallucinogenic plants in the forest. Moreover, nature still dominates man in the New World tropics, and one does not simply make unwanted manifestations of nature go away. Vegetable life grows so fast on this part of the planet that a cleared area is overgrown again in a few weeks if not constantly tended. The Indians who live in this plant-dominated world wisely choose not to fight nature's tendency to shower them with hallucinogens. Instead, they have explored the alternative of trying to make these plants work for them—to incorporate their use into society in beneficial ways.

I consider it most significant that these Indians use drugs in natural forms. They often prepare natural substances in elaborate ways; for example, the resin that goes into *epená* is concentrated by boiling and mixed with inert ingredients to produce the final snuff. But they do not attempt to refine these substances into pure, potent forms or to extract active principles from natural drugs. By contrast, most of the drugs in use in our society—aside from wine and beer, caffeine beverages, tobacco, marijuana, and occasional peyote—are highly refined, often synthetic chemicals.

It is a striking empirical fact that the difficulties individuals and societies get into with drugs appear to be correlated with the purity or potency of substances in use: the more potent the drugs, the more trouble associated with them. Opium forms a relatively harmless habit in that a high percentage of users can smoke it for years without developing troublesome problems with tolerance. Dependence on opium, if stable, can be as consistent with social productivity as dependence on coffee or tobacco. But when morphine, the active principle of opium, is isolated and made available, problems do appear. In particular, a significant percentage of users (though possibly still a minority) finds it impossible to achieve equilibrium with habitual use of morphine or with the still more potent derivative, heroin, and these unstable users eventually behave in socially disruptive ways. The same kinds of comparisons can be made between coca leaf and cocaine, peyote and mescaline, the "magic mushrooms" of Mexico and psilocybin. In all cases, the more potent forms are associated with more problems. The same trend is obvious in comparisons of societies that use different forms of alcohol. The kinds of alcoholism are worse and the numbers of people affected greater in countries like Norway and Sweden where distilled liquors are preferred than in countries like Italy where wine and beer predominate.

In addition, there is great logic behind the supposition that natural forms of drugs are inherently less dangerous than derived products. Plants that trigger altered states of consciousness never contain just one chemical. Usually, they contain a host of related compounds, all of which contribute to the pharmacological action of the whole plant.

Opium, for example, contains twenty-one alkaloids besides morphine. Peyote has at least a score of alkaloids of which mescaline is just one. Now, it is true that one compound can often be identified as the principal constituent in that it reproduces most of the action of the whole plant, but it seems to me a most unhelpful way of thinking to call this compound the active principle and to dismiss all the rest as inactive. It is also true that the other compounds may do little when administered to subjects in isolated fashion. (For example, the inactive alkaloids of peyote may cause nothing more than nausea and dizziness if taken in pure form.) But this observation does not mean that these other constituents are inactive in the whole plant. Their action is to modify the action of the dominant constituent: to play down some of its effects, to enhance others, much as harmonic overtones modify the sound of a pure tone to produce the distinctive timbre of a musical instrument. Ethyl butyrate, the pure chemical ester that is the principal component of an artificial strawberry flavoring, could be described as the active principle of that fruit, but to my mind there is a world of difference between it and the natural taste of strawberries.

Yet modern pharmacologists work on the assumption that pure active principles are equivalent to complex natural drugs. Thus they study cocaine instead of coca, mescaline instead of peyote, psilocybin instead of magic mushrooms, and now THC (tetrahydrocannabinol) instead of marijuana. During our marijuana experiments in Boston, Norman Zinberg and I were under pressure by pharmacologists to use THC rather than marijuana to make our studies more "meaningful." [Dr. Zinberg is associate professor of clinical psychiatry at the Harvard Medical School.—Eds.] And much of the research now being funded by NIMH [National Institute of Mental Health] is using pure THC (often administered orally) rather than the natural drug. Pharmacologists cling to this way of thinking because they imagine pure compounds give better results. What they mean is that lab-

oratory studies can be designed more rigorously if one ad-
ministers exact doses of single compounds. But if experimental rigor is obtained at the expense of relevance to the
world beyond the laboratory, it is not desirable. People do
not eat THC outside of laboratories; they smoke marijuana.
The subjective experience of smoking marijuana is not the
same as the subjective experience of eating (or smoking)
THC. Similarly, mescaline is not peyote, cocaine is not coca,
morphine is not opium. And, in view of the observation that
potent derivatives cause far more trouble to human beings
than natural forms of drugs, these differences seem very
much worth respecting. I have already mentioned the sym-
metries in thinking one can see between drug abusers and
drug researchers; I think it is no accident that both groups in
our society prefer to use pure, potent chemicals rather than
substances in the forms given to us by nature. And I consider
the Indians' preference for natural drugs one reason why
they do not have a drug problem.

Another reason, perhaps a more important one, is that
they recognize the normality of the human drive to experience altered states of consciousness periodically and the
prominence of the drive in growing children. Rather than
try to thwart the expression of this need, the Indians choose
to introduce children to these experiences by letting them
try drugs under supervision. Supervision is provided by the
tribal expert in such matters, usually the witch doctor. It
is noteworthy that the witch doctor is a drug expert solely
by virtue of his own experience; because of his familiarity
with states of consciousness induced by drugs he is considered qualified to guide others through these experiences.

Furthermore, the use of drugs in Indian societies is highly
ritualized. That is, drugs are taken in certain ways for certain purposes. Some drugs are used only by witch doctors
for purposes of divination or diagnosing of illness. For
example, the witch doctor might take a drug and sit with his
patient; while in an altered state of consciousness, he would
attempt to commune with the spirit world in order to learn

the nature of the disease. Other drugs, like the *ayahuasca* of certain Peruvian tribes, are used by adolescent males in coming-of-age rites. Still others, like the *epená* of the Waiká, are used as recreational intoxicants, and recreation is recognized as a legitimate purpose for altering consciousness. All of these uses are surrounded by ritual: at every step of the process, from cutting the plants to administering the prepared drugs, the Indians do things in traditional, careful, often elaborate ways, even when use appears to be casual, as in the case of the Waikás and their *epená* snuff.

This kind of ritual seems to protect individuals and groups from the negative effects of drugs, possibly by establishing a framework of order around their use. At least, people who use drugs ritually tend not to get into trouble with them, whereas people who abandon ritual and use drugs wantonly tend to have problems. We can see this protective function of ritual in our own society with our uses of alcohol. Americans who lay down a ritual for drinking—for example, people who drink only after 6 P.M., only with others present, only with food present, and only for a specified period before supper for the purpose of promoting social intercourse—are not the people who get into trouble with alcohol. Americans who get into trouble with alcohol are those who begin to use it without ritualistic rules and forms; uncontained by ritual, their drug abuse becomes unstable and begins to disrupt their lives.

I see the same principle at work among people I know who use marijuana. Those who use it ritually—that is, in groups as a recreational intoxicant or before going to a movie or before eating a good meal—do not have their lives taken over by their drug use. But those who dispense with ritual and smoke marijuana whenever they feel like it begin to get into a worse and worse relationship with the drug. I remember also that when I lived and worked in the Haight-Ashbury district of San Francisco, the people I met who were in the very worst relationships with drugs (usually with amphetamines, barbiturates, alcohol, and heroin) were always the people who had done away with rules entirely and used drugs according to no logical plan.

Probably, the effectiveness of ritual is independent of its content. I do not think it matters much what rules one makes for using drugs as long as one makes rules. If a rationale is needed for these rules, any rationale will do as long as it is consistent with prevailing beliefs. In Indian societies ritual is often explained in terms of respect for the god or spirit supposed to dwell within the magic plant. In American society, ritual may be understood as "good social form." In either case, the principle works to protect users from the negative potential of drugs.

One aspect of Indian ritual that deserves special emphasis is the use of altered states of consciousness for positive ends. That is, drug-induced states are not entered for negative reasons (such as escape from boredom or anxiety); rather, they are entered because they can be of positive usefulness to individuals and the tribe. I stress this point because it contrasts sharply with practices in the United States. Very many Americans take drugs for negative reasons or no reasons at all, and, again, I suspect this difference is a key factor in our having a drug problem. The principle that positive application of altered consciousness is protective is apparent among amphetamine users in our country. . . . The people who . . . get into trouble with amphetamines are those who begin to take them just because they like the feeling of stimulation. Just liking the feelings drugs provide without using those feelings for positive purposes seems to me to be the beginning of most bad relationships with drugs—that is, patterns of use destined to become more and more unstable and more and more dominating of the user's life. . . .

These observations are further evidence that the "magic" of drugs resides within the mind of the user, not in the drugs —a principle the Indians do not seem to have grasped. Most tribes that alter consciousness by chemical means protect themselves from this disruptive potential of drugs by using natural substances, by educating children in their "right" use, by surrounding the process with ritual, and by applying the altered states of consciousness to positive ends for the general welfare. But they tend not to realize that the experiences can be had without the drugs. Rather, they consider the plant sources of their intoxicants magical—the dwelling places of gods or spirits that transport the user to divine realms when they enter the body. Consistent with this view is the tendency of Indians to use drugs that produce considerable pharmacological noise. *Ayahuasca, epená,* and, certainly, the peyote of North American Indians all have powerful effects on the physical nervous system. In Indian societies, set and setting strongly encourage individuals to interpret these effects as preludes to intense, desired states of consciousness. By contrast, non-Indians who try these drugs, even in the same settings, often experience these same effects as symptoms of physical illness.

IV. PERSONAL ACCOUNTS

EDITORS' INTRODUCTION

Since any experience with drugs is a private, subjective one, personal accounts of drug taking are highly valuable for their revealing insights.

The first autobiographical note in this section is by the jazz musician Mezz Mezzrow, who recounts his first experience with marijuana. Drugs, as even the public has been aware, have always been part of the world of jazz because of the belief of many jazz musicians that drugs improve their music (a claim disputed by Dr. David P. Ausubel in the opening selection in this book).

The second article is by the noted British novelist Aldous Huxley, who describes his first experience with mescaline, which he used, as Amazonian Indians do, for mystical purposes.

The American writer William Burroughs, on the other hand, discusses in sordid detail the horrors of his own heroin addiction and the squalid life that accompanied it. But he also tells about a little-known cure that worked for him, after everything else he had heard of and tried had failed.

The fourth account is from an Alcoholics Anonymous pamphlet. The narrator (most accounts are given orally at A.A. meetings) is a young woman who began drinking at the age of thirteen, almost immediately got into trouble with alcohol, and joined A.A. at the age of sixteen. The next article in this section is a highly personal report by the caricaturist Al Hirschfeld on the trials and tribulations of trying to stop smoking.

The last article recounts a public-spirited, self-inflicted experiment conducted by a disc jockey on his afternoon radio show on July 4, 1974. Consuming a fifth of Scotch whisky during a four-hour period, while he was on the air, he gave a vivid first-hand demonstration of the effects of liquor in an effort to discourage holiday drivers from drinking.

MARIJUANA [1]

As soon as we were alone he [a jockey named Patrick] pulled out a gang of cigarettes and handed them to me. They were as fat as ordinary cigarettes but were rolled in brown wheatstraw paper. We both lit up and I got halfway through mine, hoping they would break the news to mother gently, before he stopped me. "Hey," he said, "take it easy, kid. You want to knock yourself out?"

I didn't feel a thing and I told him so. "Do you know one thing?" he said. "You ain't even smokin' it right. You got to hold that muggle so that it barely touches your lips, see, then draw in air around it. Say *tfff, tfff,* only breathe in when you say it. Then don't blow it out right away, you got to give the stuff a chance." He had a tricky look in his eye that I didn't go for at all. The last time I saw that kind of look it was on a district attorney's mug, and it caused me a lot of inconvenience.

After I finished the weed I went back to the bandstand. Everything seemed normal and I began to play as usual. I passed a stick of gauge around for the other boys to smoke, and we started a set.

The first thing I noticed was that I began to hear my saxophone as though it was inside my head, but I couldn't hear much of the band in back of me, although I knew they were there. All the other instruments sounded like they were way off in the distance; I got the same sensation you'd get if you stuffed your ears with cotton and talked out loud. Then

[1] From the book *Really the Blues,* by Milton ("Mezz") Mezzrow and Bernard Wolfe. Random House. '46. p 71-7. Copyright 1946 by Milton Mezzrow and Bernard Wolfe. Copyright renewed, 1973. Reprinted by permission of Harold Matson Company, Inc. "Mezz" Mezzrow (1899-1972), a noted white jazz musician, for a time sold marijuana in Harlem and received a three-year prison sentence for possession of marijuana. Bernard Wolfe is a professional writer.

I began to feel the vibrations of the reed much more pronounced against my lip, and my head buzzed like a loudspeaker. I found I was slurring much better and putting just the right feeling into my phrases—I was really coming on. All the notes came easing out of my horn like they'd already been made up, greased and stuffed into the bell, so all I had to do was blow a little and send them on their way, one right after the other, never missing, never behind time, all without an ounce of effort. The phrases seemed to have more continuity to them and I was sticking to the theme without ever going tangent. I felt I could go on playing for years without running out of ideas and energy. There wasn't any struggle; it was all made-to-order and suddenly there wasn't a sour note or a discord in the world that could bother me. I began to feel very happy and sure of myself. With my loaded horn I could take all the fist-swinging, evil things in the world and bring them together in perfect harmony, spreading peace and joy and relaxation to all the keyed-up and punchy people everywhere. I began to preach my millenniums on my horn, leading all the sinners on to glory. . . .

It's a funny thing about marijuana—when you first begin smoking it you see things in a wonderful soothing, easygoing new light. All of a sudden the world is stripped of its dirty gray shrouds and becomes one big bellyful of giggles, a spherical laugh, bathed in brilliant, sparkling colors that hit you like a heatwave. Nothing leaves you cold any more; there's a humorous tickle and great meaning in the least little thing, the twitch of somebody's little finger or the click of a beer glass. All your pores open like funnels, your nerve-ends stretch their mouths wide, hungry and thirsty for new sights and sounds and sensations; and every sensation, when it comes, is the most exciting one you've ever had. You can't get enough of anything—you want to gobble up the whole goddamned universe just for an appetizer. Them first kicks are a killer, Jim.

Suppose you're the critical and analytical type, always

ripping things to pieces, tearing the covers off and being disgusted by what you find under the sheet. Well, under the influence of muta [marijuana] you don't lose your surgical touch exactly, but you don't come up evil and grimy about it. You still see what you saw before but in a different, more tolerant way, through rose-colored glasses, and things that would have irritated you before just tickle you. Everything is good for a laugh; the wrinkles get ironed out of your face and you forget what a frown is, you just want to hold on to your belly and roar till the tears come. . . .

Tea puts a musician in a real masterly sphere, and that's why so many jazzmen have used it. You look down on the other members of the band like an old mother hen surveying her brood of chicks; if one of them hits a sour note or comes up with a bad modulation, you just smile tolerantly and figure, oh well, he'll learn, it'll be better next time, give the guy a chance. Pretty soon you find yourself helping him out, trying to put him on the right track. The most terrific thing is this, that all the while you're playing, really getting off, your own accompaniment keeps flashing through your head, just like you were a one-man band. You hear the basic tones of the theme and keep up your pattern of improvisation without ever getting tangled up, giving out with a uniform sequence all the way. Nothing can mess you up. You hear everything at once and you hear it right. When you get that feeling of power and sureness, you're in a solid groove.

You know how jittery, got-to-be-moving people in the city always get up in the subway train two minutes before they arrive at the station? Their nerves are on edge; they're watching the clock, thinking about schedules, full of that high-powered mile-a-minute jive. Well, when you've picked up on some gauge that clock just stretches its arms, yawns, and dozes off. The whole world slows down and gets drowsy. You wait until the train stops dead and the doors slide open, then you get up and stroll out in slow motion, like a sleep-walker with a long night ahead of him and no appointments to keep. You've got all the time in the world. What's the rush, buddy? Take-it-easy, that's the play, it's bound to sweeten it all the way. . . .

The bandstand was only a foot high but when I went to step down it took me a year to find the floor, it seemed so far away. I was sailing through the clouds, flapping my free-wheeling wings, and leaving the stand was like stepping off into space. Twelve months later my foot struck solid ground with a jolt, but the other one stayed up there on those lovely soft clouds, and I almost fell flat on my face. There was a roar of laughter from Patrick's table and I began to feel self-conscious and nauseous at the same time. I flew to the men's room and got there just in time. Patrick came in and started to laugh at me.

"What's the matter, kid?" he said. "You not feeling so good?" At that moment I was up in a plane, soaring around the sky, with a buzz-saw in my head. Up and around we went, saying nuts to Newton and all his fancy laws of gravitation, but suddenly we went into a nosedive and I came down to earth, sock. Ouch. My head went spattering off in more directions than a hand grenade. Patrick put a cold towel on my temples and I snapped out of it. After sitting down for a while I was all right.

When I went back to the stand I still heard all my music amplified, as though my ear was built right into the horn. The evening rolled away before I knew it. When the entertainers sang I accompanied them on the piano, and from the way they kept glancing up at me I could tell they felt the harmonies I was inventing behind them without any effort at all. The notes kept sliding out of my horn like bubbles in seltzer water. My control over the vibrations of my tones was perfect, and I got a terrific lift from the richness of the music, the bigness of it. The notes eased out like lava running down a mountain, slow and sure and steaming. It was good.

MESCALINE [2]

Most takers of mescaline experience only the heavenly part of schizophrenia. The drug brings hell and purgatory only to those who have had a recent case of jaundice, or who suffer from periodical depressions or a chronic anxiety. If, like the other drugs of remotely comparable power, mescaline were notoriously toxic, the taking of it would be enough, of itself, to cause anxiety. But the reasonably healthy person knows in advance that, so far as he is concerned, mescaline is completely innocuous, that its effects will pass off after eight or ten hours, leaving no hangover and consequently no craving for a renewal of the dose. Fortified by this knowledge, he embarks upon the experiment without fear—in other words, without any disposition to convert an unprecedentedly strange and other than human experience into something appalling, something actually diabolical.

Confronted by a chair which looked like the Last Judgment—or, to be more accurate, by a Last Judgment which, after a long time and with considerable difficulty, I recognized as a chair—I found myself all at once on the brink of panic. This, I suddenly felt, was going too far. Too far, even though the going was into intenser beauty, deeper significance. The fear, as I analyze it in retrospect, was of being overwhelmed, of disintegrating under a pressure of reality greater than a mind, accustomed to living most of the time in a cosy world of symbols, could possibly bear. . . .

None too soon, I was steered away from the disquieting splendors of my garden chair. Drooping in green parabolas from the hedge, the ivy fronds shone with a kind of glassy, jade-like radiance. A moment later a clump of Red Hot

[2] From *The Doors of Perception*, by Aldous Huxley (1894–1963), British novelist and essayist greatly interested in mind-altering drugs and visionary experiences. Harper. '54. Abridged from p 54-62 in *The Doors of Perception and Heaven and Hell*, by Aldous Huxley. Copyright 1954 by Aldous Huxley. By permission of Harper & Row, Publishers, Inc.

Pokers, in full bloom, had exploded into my field of vision.
So passionately alive that they seemed to be standing on the
very brink of utterance, the flowers strained upwards into
the blue. Like the chair under the laths, they protected too
much. I looked down at the leaves and discovered a cavern-
ous intricacy of the most delicate green lights and shadows,
pulsing with undecipherable mystery.

> Roses:
> The flowers are easy to paint,
> The leaves difficult.

Shiki's *haiku* (which I quote in R. H. Blyth's translation)
expresses, by indirection, exactly what I then felt—the excessive, the too obvious glory of the flowers, as contrasted
with the subtler miracle of their foliage.

We walked out into the street. A large pale blue automobile was standing at the curb. At the sight of it, I was
suddenly overcome by enormous merriment. What com-
placency, what an absurd self-satisfaction beamed from those
bulging surfaces of glossiest enamel! Man had created the
thing in his own image—or rather in the image of his fa-
vorite character in fiction. I laughed till the tears ran down
my cheeks.

We reentered the house. A meal had been prepared.
Somebody, who was not yet identical with myself, fell to
with ravenous appetite. From a considerable distance and
without much interest, I looked on.

When the meal had been eaten, we got into the car and
went for a drive. The effects of the mescaline were already
on the decline: but the flowers in the gardens still trembled
on the brink of being supernatural, the pepper trees and
carobs along the side streets still manifestly belonged to
some sacred grove. Eden alternated with Dodona. Yggdrasil
with the mystic Rose. And then, abruptly, we were at an
intersection, waiting to cross Sunset Boulevard. Before us the
cars were rolling by in a steady stream—thousands of them,
all bright and shiny like an advertiser's dream and each

more ludicrous than the last. Once again I was convulsed with laughter.

The Red Sea of traffic parted at last, and we crossed into another oasis of trees and lawns and roses. In a few minutes we had climbed to a vantage point in the hills, and there was the city spread out beneath us. Rather disappointingly, it looked very like the city I had seen on other occasions. So far as I was concerned, transfiguration was proportional to distance. The nearer, the more divinely other. This vast, dim panorama was hardly different from itself. . . .

An hour later, with ten more miles and the visit to the World's Biggest Drug Store safely behind us, we were back at home, and I had returned to that reassuring but profoundly unsatisfactory state known as "being in one's right mind."

HEROIN [3]

I awoke from The Sickness at the age of forty-five, calm and sane, and in reasonably good health except for a weakened liver and the look of borrowed flesh common to all who survive The Sickness. . . . Most survivors do not remember the delirium in detail. I apparently took detailed notes on sickness and delirium. I have no precise memory of writing the notes which have now been published under the title *Naked Lunch*. The title was suggested by Jack Kerouac. I did not understand what the title meant until my recent recovery. The title means exactly what the words say: NAKED Lunch—a frozen moment when everyone sees what is on the end of every fork.

The Sickness is drug addiction and I was an addict for fifteen years. When I say addict I mean an addict to *junk* (generic term for opium and/or derivatives including all synthetics from demerol to palfium). I have used junk in

[3] Excerpts from "Deposition: Testimony Concerning a Sickness," by William Burroughs, novelist, author of *Junkie. Evergreen Review.* No. 11:15-22. Ja/F. '60. Reprinted by permission of Grove Press, Inc. Copyright © 1960.

many forms: morphine, heroin, dilaudid, eukodal, panta-
pon, diocodid, diosane, opium, demerol, dolophine, palfium.
I have smoked junk, eaten it, sniffed it, injected it in vein-
skin-muscle, inserted it in rectal suppositories. The needle is
not important. Whether you sniff it smoke it eat it . . . the
result is the same: addiction. When I speak of drug addiction I do not refer to keif, marijuana or any preparation of
hashish, mescaline, Bannisteria Caapi, LSD6, Sacred Mushrooms or any other drug of the hallucinogen group. . . .
There is no evidence that the use of any hallucinogen results
in physical dependence. The action of these drugs is physio-
logically opposite to the action of junk. A lamentable confusion between the two classes of drugs has arisen owing to
the zeal of the US and other narcotic departments.

I have seen the exact manner in which the junk virus
operates through fifteen years of addiction. The pyramid of
junk, one level eating the level below (it is no accident that
junk higher-ups are always fat and the addict in the street is
always thin) right up to the top or tops since there are many
junk pyramids feeding on peoples of the world and all built
on basic principles of monopoly:

1. Never give anything away for nothing.
2. Never give more than you have to give (always catch
   the buyer hungry and always make him wait).
3. Always take everything back if you possibly can.

The Pusher always gets it all back. The addict needs more
and more junk to maintain a human form . . . buy off the
Monkey.

Junk is the mold of monopoly and possession. The addict
stands by while his junk legs carry him straight in on the
junk beam to relapse. Junk is quantitative and accurately
measurable. The more junk you use the less you have and
the more you have the more you use. All the hallucinogen
drugs are considered sacred by those who use them—there
are peyote cults and Bannisteria cults, hashish cults and
mushroom cults—"the Sacred Mushrooms of Mexico enable
a man to see God"—but no one ever suggested that junk is

sacred. There are no opium cults. Opium is profane and quantitative like money. I have heard that there was once a beneficent non-habit-forming junk in India. It was called *soma* and is pictured as a beautiful blue tide. If *soma* ever existed the Pusher was there to bottle it and monopolize it and sell it and it turned into plain old time JUNK.

Junk is the ideal product . . . the ultimate merchandise. No sales talk necessary. The client will crawl through a sewer and beg to buy. . . . The junk merchant does not sell his product to the consumer, he sells the consumer to his product. He does not improve and simplify his merchandise. He degrades and simplifies the client. He pays his staff in junk.

Junk yields a basic formula of "evil" virus: *The Algebra of Need.* The face of "evil" is always the face of total need. A dope fiend is a man in total need of dope. Beyond a certain frequency need knows absolutely no limit or control. In the words of total need: *"Wouldn't you?"* Yes you would. You would lie, cheat, inform on your friends, steal, do *anything* to satisfy total need. Because you would be in a state of total sickness, total possession, and not in a position to act in any other way. Dope fiends are sick people who cannot act other than they do. A rabid dog cannot choose but bite. . . .

If you wish to alter or annihilate a pyramid of numbers in a serial relation, you alter or remove the bottom number. If we wish to annihilate the junk pyramid, we must start with the bottom of the pyramid: the Addict in the Street, and stop tilting quixotically for the "higher ups" so called, all of whom are immediately replaceable. The addict in the street who must have junk to live is the one irreplaceable factor in the junk equation. When there are no more addicts to buy junk there will be no junk traffic. As long as junk need exists, someone will service it.

Addicts can be cured or quarantined—that is allowed a morphine ration under minimal supervision like typhoid carriers. When this is done, junk pyramids of the world will collapse. So far as I know, England is the only country to apply this method to the junk problem. They have about five hundred quarantined addicts in the UK. In another generation when the quarantined addicts die off and pain killers operating on a nonjunk principle are discovered, the junk virus will be like smallpox, a closed chapter—a medical curiosity.

The vaccine that can relegate the junk virus to a land-locked past is in existence. This vaccine is the apomorphine treatment discovered by an English doctor whose name I must withhold pending his permission to use it and to quote from his book covering thirty years of apomorphine treatment of addicts and alcoholics. The compound apomorphine is formed by boiling morphine with hydrochloric acid. It was discovered years before it was used to treat addicts. For many years the only use for apomorphine which has no narcotic or pain-killing properties was an emetic to induce vomiting in cases of poisoning. It acts directly on the vomiting center in the back brain.

I found this vaccine at the end of the junk line. I lived in one room in the native quarter of Tangier. I had not taken a bath in a year nor changed my clothes or removed them except to stick a needle every hour in the fibrous grey wooden flesh of terminal addiction. I never cleaned or dusted the room. Empty ampule boxes and garbage piled to the ceiling. Light and water long since turned off for nonpayment. I did absolutely nothing. I could look at the end of my shoe for eight hours. I was only roused to action when the hourglass of junk ran out. If a friend came to visit—and they rarely did since who or what was left to visit—I sat there not caring that he had entered my field of vision—a grey screen always blanker and fainter—and not caring when he walked out of it. If he had died on the spot I would have sat there looking at my shoe waiting to go through his pockets. Wouldn't you? Because I never had enough junk—no one ever does. Thirty grains of morphine a day and it still was not enough. And long waits in front of the drugstore. Delay is a rule in the junk business. The Man is never on time. This is no accident. There are no accidents in the junk world. The addict is taught again and again exactly what will happen if he does not score for his junk ration. Get up that money or else. And suddenly my habit began to jump and jump. Forty, sixty grains a day. And it still was not enough. And I could not pay.

I stood there with my last check in my hand and realized that it was my last check. I took the next plane for London.

The doctor explained to me that apomorphine acts on the back brain to regulate the metabolism and normalize the blood stream in such a way that the enzyme system of addiction is destroyed over a period of four or five days. Once the back brain is regulated apomorphine can be discontinued and only used in case of relapse. (No one would take apomorphine for kicks. *Not one case of addiction to apomorphine has ever been recorded.*) I agreed to undergo treatment and entered a nursing home. For the first twenty-four hours I was literally insane and paranoid as many addicts are in severe withdrawal. This delirium was dispersed by twenty-four hours of intensive apomorphine treatment. The doctor showed me the chart. I had received minute amounts of morphine that could not possibly account for my lack of the more severe withdrawal symptoms such as leg and stomach cramps, fever and my own special symptom, The Cold Burn, like a vast hive covering the body and rubbed with menthol. Every addict has his own special symptom that cracks all control. There was a missing factor in the withdrawal equation—that factor could only be apomorphine.

I saw the apomorphine treatment really work. Eight days later I left the nursing home eating and sleeping normally. I remained completely off junk for two full years—a twelve-year record. I did relapse for some months as a result of pain and illness. Another apomorphine cure has kept me off junk through this writing.

The apomorphine cure is qualitatively different from

other methods of cure. I have tried them all. Short reduction, slow reduction, cortisone, antihistamines, tranquilizers,
sleeping cures, tolserol, reserpine. None of these cures lasted
beyond the first opportunity to relapse. I can say definitely
that I was never *metabolically* cured until I took the apomorphine cure. The overwhelming relapse statistics from
the Lexington Narcotic Hospital have led many doctors to
say that addiction is not curable. They use a dolophine reduction cure at Lexington and have never tried apomorphine so far as I know. In fact, this method of treatment has
been largely neglected. No research has been done with
variations of the apomorphine formula or with synthetics.
No doubt substances fifty times stronger than apomorphine
could be developed and the side effect of vomiting eliminated.

Apomorphine is a metabolic and psychic regulator that
can be discontinued as soon as it has done its work. The
world is deluged with tranquilizers and energizers but this
unique regulator has not received attention. No research has
been done by any of the large pharmaceutical companies. I
suggest that research with variations of apomorphine and
synthesis of it will open a new medical frontier extending far
beyond the problem of addiction.

The smallpox vaccine was opposed by a vociferous luna-
tic group of antivaccinationists. No doubt a scream of protest will go up from interested or unbalanced individuals as
the junk virus is shot out from under them. Junk is big business; there are always cranks and operators. They must not
be allowed to interfere with the essential work of inocula-
tion treatment and quarantine. The junk virus is public
health problem number one of the world today.

A TEENAGE ALCOHOLIC [4]

"Now I tell that crowd, 'You're full of fear, baby.' "

I tried for ages to get a date with one of the guys in the crowd. Those were the people I then considered the swingers —the ones that cruised, the girls that ran in and out of bedrooms, the guys that shot heroin and smoked dope. One of them asked me out finally, and that was the first night I got drunk, when I was thirteen. He kept switching cans from his six-pack into mine, so I drank more than he did. On the way home. I fell over towards the door to throw up out the window, and the boys shoved me out of the car and left me in the street.

The crowd didn't want me. I didn't know what was going on. Well, I intended to find out what was going on. So I learned to drink with the crowd. I practiced to be the way other people were. I sat in the kitchen and I told the dirtiest jokes and I drank the most beer.

Now, when I see some of that crowd, I tell them, "You're full of fear, baby, and that's all there is to it." People stick together because they're scared of what they really are. They never had an identity, and they stick to each other and get this big identity, and then they are scared to death to let go of it.

That's why I was a people-pleaser—not because I wanted to be one of the hard, hard girls. I put up the front, but I was never really like them. I wouldn't smoke grass, because I knew that girls that smoked it got into a lot of trouble, ending up in jail—no big thing where I live in this town. Girls twelve, thirteen, and fourteen are having babies, living in juvenile and foster homes. It's a mess! Thank God, that didn't happen to me.

I have seven brothers and sisters, and no one ever really

[4] "Rose Joined A.A. at Age 16," excerpt from *Young People and A.A.*, pamphlet published by A.A. World Services, Inc. '69. p 30-3, Copyright © 1969. Reprinted with permission of A.A. World Services, Inc., copyright owners, P.O. Box 459, Grand Central Station, New York, N.Y. 10017.

got into trouble other than me and a brother two years older. I never got along with my family, and I used to shock my mother an awful lot. I was an A student, and I did some good writing, but after I started drinking, it soon got to where I cut school. (My friends were dropping out, one by one.) I drank beer, wine, rum. I used to carry an extra-large straw purse, because I could get four quarts of whiskey in there.

One night when I was fifteen, a guy put LSD tablets in my drink. People say I snapped. For the next seven months, I was continually taking trips. I had blackouts. They would say, "That was a boss joke, Rose," and I would say, "What? Did I tell a joke?" I made four institutions. Once, a state mental hospital wouldn't accept me because I was only fifteen—and drunk and couldn't sign myself in.

The beginning of the end for me was the time I went to a motel with a gang of nine kids, and snapped, and wound up in the hospital that night. Right before my brother walked in to visit me, I'd had a fit, and the nurses had me tied down. My brother was loaded, and he turned around and drove all the way back home and found the first guy that had given me acid, and he beat up on that guy.

That is the first time I remember any kind of protection from my family. I thought it was my father's fault because I cussed so much, and my mother's fault I was sick, and my sister's fault I felt dirty inside, because of the name she called me for years. The truth was, *I* didn't like Rose—so how could anyone else like her? My family couldn't afford to care about me, because of some of the things I did. I know now that it was a sickness, and I'm not ashamed any more. Being sick is not a reason to stay sick—it's a reason to get off your backside and start getting well.

One day after I got home from the hospital, my father asked me, "Rose, what's bothering you?"

"Daddy, I'm depressed."

He said, "I know a place where maybe they can help you if you would like to go."

My father has been in A.A., sober, for ten years. So I went to my first A.A. meeting with him. I was shaky and scared and I couldn't understand the smiles. But the people told me, "Rose, look, we love you." No one had ever said that to me except when they had their hands on my body. I found out what love is. Love, to me, is caring because people are themselves, accepting them whether they are good, bad, or indifferent.

After that, I'd make a Sunday-morning meeting and maybe two or three meetings a week with my father. But I don't remember wanting to be sober. I would be at home and know everyone else was out getting loaded and having a good time. My last blackout, the last time I snapped on LSD, the last time I had a drink, I had been going out with a boy who was leaving for Vietnam. The night before he left, we were in a bar, and I was drinking beer. I put the glass down. "I don't know what's going to happen to anybody else," I told myself, "but I'm going to come out of this. I can't be plastered when he leaves."

I was going to see him off the next morning, but at midnight he had to bring me home. I remember lying on the bed crying, and I shook all over for about four hours. My father came in and said, "You know, the world is not ending."

I had just made a halfway stab at A.A. But now I knew I didn't want to be on the outside again. I wanted A.A. It was my last resort. That was eleven and a half months ago. A.A. has made me able to decrease my depressions. When I am hurting most, I still know if I had alcohol and drugs on top of that depression, I would be dead. I have called A.A. people at two and three in the morning. "It's going to be all right," they say, and I fall asleep talking on the telephone.

One night at an A.A. meeting, a man said to me, "Little girl, I've spilt more booze on my tie than you ever drank. Aren't you a little young to be an alcholic?"

I said, "Aren't you a little old?"

But when an old man stands in front of a meeting talking and says, "My guts hurt," my heart goes out to him, because I know how he feels. I remember lying in my bed in the hospital for days at a time, not eating. I wasn't really as dirty as a wino, but I felt the same. I felt the same! I could grab a lot of people in A.A. and put my arms around them and never let them go, especially the ones that are sick and hurt. It's good for me, because today I have a little bit of room inside me to hurt for somebody else. It's not all *me* any more.

I used to let people affect me too much—the wrong way. I've had to learn a kind of detachment. At first, I had dreams about my brother joining A.A., too. But now I am accepting the fact that he's got to live his own life. There is a place for him in A.A. if he wants it, but I am detached to the extent that I am not shoving it down his throat.

During the summer I worked as a counter girl, and now I'm back in school. My grades are better—three B's on my last report card. But I have to study and apply myself, because my mind deteriorated from just three years of drinking and using drugs. People ask me, "What do you do for fun?" I live! And I know I'm alive. It's not all good, but I don't have to run away from everything any more. I don't do the things I did when I was drinking—because I don't have to prove myself any more.

HOW I STOPPED SMOKING [5]

I have always smoked. It never occurred to me that life was possible without a pipe, cigar, hookah, cubeb or cornsilk, hand-rolled or manufactured cigarette projecting from the front of my face. And I always assumed that smoking, like pregnancy, was a matter of nature's capricious selection. One either was, or was not, a smoker: and that was that. But coughing was a different department. Coughing seemed an acquired habit. I could have sworn under oath that I

[5] From article by Al Hirschfeld, caricaturist. *Esquire.* 39:74-5. Je. '53. Reprinted by permission of *Esquire* Magazine © 1953 by Esquire, Inc.

used the cough as a social mannerism, in place of words, to cover acute cases of embarrassment. I am not referring to the common cold or virus type of cough; but to the controlled enforced jet genus, which usually accompanies a hearty laugh. They sort of go together socially. As a matter of fact, I established a considerable reputation as a raconteur based on nothing more than a well-timed combination of cough and laugh. Then, quite suddenly, the thing got out of control: my cough developed a life of its own. . . .

With each passing year it became more arrogant. My family grew accustomed to Daddy's catarrh in the middle of the night; I accepted as normal the coughing fit which attacked me every morning the moment I got out of bed and stood upright; the hysterical stagger to the bathroom gasping for breath; the clutching at the sink for support while a face, the color of an eggplant—and just about as interesting—coughed back at me in the mirror. I consoled myself with the notion that none of us was getting any younger, serves me right for sleeping on my left side, that's the last time I go to bed sober: these and similar justifications made it possible for me to live in the same house with myself.

But this insane state of affairs could not last forever, and it changed completely about three months ago, when a short, unexpected, fast cough caught me off-balance and threw me down a flight of stairs. While the doctor from the emergency ambulance was basting my calf I let go with a whopper that blew his glasses off and smashed them against the farthest wall. Retrieving the frames from the floor, he started to expostulate; then another blast stopped him short and spun his toupee around. The doctor threw up his arms in a lightning thrust to ward off another attack.

"Better take care of that cough, m'boy!" he said.

I assured him that I had tried every known cure, pill, opiate and cough medicine extant, that I had been coughing for years in every country and climate of the world, and that quite obviously there was nothing anyone could do about it.

"Ever try to give up smoking?" he said unsympathetically.

"Be easier to give up eating," I told him.

He was unimpressed. "Start tomorrow morning," he advised. "Set your alarm for ten o'clock, and no matter what happens don't take a cigarette until you hear the alarm ring; then smoke as you normally would for the rest of the day."

I promised him that I would try his system. "Keep it up for a week," he continued, "then increase the time one hour weekly. At the end of four weeks you'll suddenly discover that you've gone without a cigarette up till one o'clock in the afternoon. After that, it's easy sailing. Eat peppermints or chew gum to satisfy any temporary nervousness. The important thing is, don't cheat: remember—it's your life you're playing with."

It all sounded so crisp and easy I decided to give it a try. I have always been a sucker for reasonable advice. The only positive lesson I learned in art school was a piece of advice given me by my instructor: "Don't let the point of your pencil interfere with your artistic ability." And to this very day I cannot draw unless the point of my pencil is needle-sharp. Who knows, perhaps this strange doctor would have as profound an influence on my health as Mr. Shapiro —of the Vocational School for Boys—had on my art.

The following morning, at ten o'clock sharp, my alarm clock rang and woke me: I reached out of bed and lit a cigarette. "Why, shucks," thought I, filling my lungs with pure, rich nicotine and coal tar, "there's nothing to it."

The second morning was a trifle more difficult: I got up before the alarm went off. For some unaccountable reason, my cough blasted me out of bed at a quarter to ten. Those fifteen minutes before the alarm rang have become permanently recorded on my unbreakable memory. I took a shower, brushed my teeth, sang the complete score of *High Jinks,* looked at the clock, rang ME 7-1212 (my clock was absolutely right: five to ten), tried getting dressed, then undressed, then dressed again, picked up *War and Peace* and read it from cover to cover (still four and a half minutes to go), thought that if I live through the day I'll organize a Smokers Anonymous, reexamined Buckminster Fuller's theory of Dymaxion Energetic Geometry—and had just about discovered the flaw when the alarm rang. It was a sound such as stout Cortez may have heard at the Pacific. With trembling, bleeding fingers I lit my beard and cigarette at the same time.

Having mastered those fifteen minutes was the toughest assignment I had ever given myself; but now I am living proof that the thing can be done, and as easily as outlined in the doctor's recipe. Furthermore, it is all absolutely true. I have not coughed once in the past week, my appetite is unbelievably ravenous and my sense of smell has become so heightened that I can now distinguish the subtle aromatic distinction between different kinds of blotting paper. I have gained twenty-two pounds, and none of my clothes fit me any more. My doctor now tells me that I shall have to lose those extra pounds; too much strain on the heart.

There is no doubt about the matter: it is much easier to give up smoking than to give up eating. I can no longer work unless my drawing table is well-stocked with platters of raw carrots, cut celery, peppermints and my daily ration of four or five packs of chewing gum. My mind, free of the nicotine drug, is clear, direct, literate: no more fuzzy abstractions, meaningless fantasies, speculative illusions. A cumulus cloud against a cerulean sky no longer challenges my interpretive powers; it automatically becomes a giant turkey on a blue plate. My abstract doodlings come out as careful academic drawings of little bloated pigs with apples stuffed in their mouths. In recent weeks I have taken to roaming the streets in the middle of the night looking for an open delicatessen. Neither rain, sleet nor hail can stop me when my stomach whispers in my ear, "Corned beef on rye." And the weather has been foul. I have had a succession of sniffles, colds, wheezes and sinus attacks. Most of all, the cough, stimulated now by germs, is threatening to return in glory.

I am convinced that I have grown a small blast furnace where my stomach used to be. Any kind of food, even the pills I take, is sufficient fuel to generate a hot-air system which circulates in my throat. I have become an ice sucker as well as a gum chewer and a peppermint eater. The chewing gum and peppermints have successfully removed the thin veneer of porcelain from my teeth so that I can no longer even part my lips without severe pain. And as for my sense of smell . . . now there is one sense I think we could all happily do without. Take it from one who can smell not only all the kitchen odors, but the Airwick as well. I am afraid that if my sense of smell improves any more I shall have to leave the city. The stink is unbearable. Equipped with these heightened senses and a new pair of spectacles—through which I cannot help seeing every hair follicle and pimple on a face a block away—I fail to see the advantage of preserving a lung or two at the expense of the stomach, heart, teeth and nervous system. As for me, I shall face the future with a stogie firmly clamped between my teeth and an unpredictable cough lurking in my throat. Happy and unafraid.

ALCOHOL ON THE AIR: A DISC JOCKEY'S EXPERIMENT [6]

Disc jockey Ted Brown took the fifth before a jury of thousands and the verdict was unanimous: Dead Drunk.

The WNEW-AM star, whose voice normally is familiar to a host of homeward bound commuters, found his tongue a little furry yesterday and his speech a little slurred as he progressively downed a fifth of Scotch during his afternoon show [on July 4, 1974].

[6] Reprint of "DJ Takes a Dizzy Spin So Drivers Won't," article by William T. Slattery, staff reporter. New York *Post*. p 4. Jl. 5, '74. Reprinted by permission of New York *Post*, © 1974, New York Post Corporation.

Watching the normally witty Brown degenerate as alcohol numbed his brain was funny—but the purpose was deadly serious.

Brown drank himself into a July the Fifth hangover to prove to holiday drivers that they should not drink and drive.

"I'm not a drinker at all," Brown said before cracking the seal on the twelve-year-old Scotch. "I've only been drunk a few times. My wife, Renee, is a little upset about this, too.

"Last year—the first year I did this—was easier," he said. "I didn't know what would happen. This year I know. I'm going to be very sick. But if I can keep one person from driving after drinking, it will be worth it."

Brown shared his Metromedia studio with Sergeants Richard Holden and Ernest Floegel of the [New York] State Police and Valerie Lezoli, supervisor of nurses at Bellevue [Hospital in New York].

Five times during the course of the four-hour show, which began at 4 P.M., the troopers tested Brown's blood for alcohol content and Miss Lezoli took his pulse and blood pressure.

The result: His heart kept beating but his brain was taking a beating:

5:25 P.M. Brown pales when informed that cirrhosis can bring on irreversible impotence.

5:47 P.M. The top-label spinner turned Black Label drinker can't hear his engineer, Laurie Richman, because his earphones are on backwards.

6 P.M. While turning the air over to the news department, he forgets the name of the radio station.

6:05 P.M. Brown walks behind Floegel, jabs a finger in his back and says, "Stick 'em up." It takes a while before Floegel smiles.

6:59 P.M. He announces to thousands, "We're going to have an on-the-air vomit."

7:15 P.M. Brown tries to call home and forgets the number.

7:25 P.M. He tries a police reaction timer and can't find the simulated brake pedal.

With only seven seconds to go, Brown finally was whisked off the air because he started to cry while thinking of his family. "He's devoted to his kids," a colleague said. "Last year he started to cry at 7:15."

Holden said that the level at which a person is legally [drunk] here is one tenth of 1 percent of alcohol in the blood. By 7:20 P.M., after nine drinks swallowed by the increasingly reluctant star, Brown's blood level was one thirteenth of 1 percent.

"I felt lousy long before this," Brown said, his normally melodious voice running the words together. "Anyone who drives when he's like this is crazy. It's like taking a gun and shooting into a crowd."

Floegel said that last year the state police made 12,305 arrests for drunk driving—3,157 of them were made after the drivers were involved in accidents.

The show featured tunes chosen by an unsympathetic coworker. As Brown grimaced and tossed down a shot, he played "The Days of Wine and Roses," "Kisses Sweeter than Wine" and "My Cup Runneth Over."

V. POSSIBLE SOLUTIONS

EDITORS' INTRODUCTION

The articles comprising the final section of this book discuss some of the approaches now being used to deal constructively with the drug situation in America.

The first three articles concern methadone. Pioneers in the development of methadone maintenance programs were Dr. Vincent P. Dole, a specialist in metabolic diseases, and Dr. Marie Nyswander, a psychiatrist. Methadone, however, though one of the most useful substances thus far developed for the treatment of heroin and morphine addiction, is itself addictive and therefore controversial.

The fourth selection is the basic credo of Alcoholics Anonymous—the Twelve Steps—upon which much of the organization's valuable work is based.

The extracts that follow, from *Licit and Illicit Drugs,* go together as a unit. The subject is the youth subculture: its historical context, the reasons for the specific nature of this subculture at this time, and the members' own methods for dealing with their problems.

The final article is the only one in this compilation to deal with the subject of adolescent problems from the point of view of parents. Actually, the author uses a massive middle-class drug arrest as a point of departure to discuss positive parental attitudes towards near-adult sons and daughters. So, strictly speaking, "Welcome to the Club" is not about drugs, but rather about growing up in general.

METHADONE [1]

Methadone is a narcotic, yet it has become one of the most useful treatments for morphine and heroin addiction.

[1] Excerpt from *The Television Report: Drugs, A to Z,* by Earl Ubell. WCBS-TV. 51 W. 52d St. New York 10019. '70. Reprinted with permission from WCBS-TV and the author.

Medically, the Germans first used methadone in World War I as a painkiller. Because it differed chemically from morphine they hoped methadone was not addictive, but unfortunately it was.

Then in the 1950s scientists discovered that methadone could help bring an addict of heroin or morphine off his drug without withdrawal symptoms. In the 1960s they discovered that a person receiving methadone periodically in small doses would not get high if he then took heroin or morphine. Methadone blocks the action of either drug. And thus began the controversial methadone maintenance program. So far, many addicts sustained with methadone, which they take in a cup of orange juice, do go back to work and restore near-normal human relationships. It doesn't seem to work for the person who was a bad social risk before he became a narcotics addict.

Critics of the program claim that methadone maintenance programs substitute one narcotic for another. They warn that addicts may have to take methadone for life and they assert that individuals do get high on methadone and still take other drugs. The supporters of the methadone program say that each criticism may be true in part. But they say that their program is the only one that consistently keeps heroin and morphine addicts off their drugs.

Other Treatments

There are other drug treatments. One is cyclazocine and the other, brand new, is called naloxone. Both antagonize heroin or morphine. If you give a shot of either cyclazocine or naloxone to an addict, he immediately goes into withdrawal symptoms. But if the addict is already clean, a small dose of either cyclazocine or naloxone taken by mouth will prevent the addict from receiving any sort of reaction if he takes either heroin or morphine. Doctors now plan to give small daily doses of either cyclazocine or naloxone to addicts by mouth. And that means when they return to the drug scene and are pressured into taking a narcotic, they'll get no high from it; that is, they won't get the psychological reward and, therefore, addiction will not be reestablished. So far, however, neither drug has been tried on a wide scale.

WHY METHADONE MAINTENANCE WORKS [2]

The two major reasons for the success of methadone maintenance are surely no secret. Methadone is legal; hence the addict who enters a methadone maintenance program casts off his role of hated and hunted criminal when he downs his first methadone tablet or glass of methadone-spiked orange drink. And methadone is cheap. The cost of the usual dose—100 milligrams per day—is ten cents. It is supplied the addict either free or (in some programs with ancillary services outside New York) for $10 to $14 per week.

If morphine or heroin were legally dispensed at low cost, the same two advantages would be equally well achieved. Thus in those two respects the favorable results of methadone maintenance cannot be attributed solely to the methadone.

Like morphine and heroin, methadone is a narcotic and therefore, by definition, an addicting drug. This fact is often cited as a disadvantage. Indeed, newspapers, politicians, and even some physicians have expressed the hope that a non-addicting drug for the treatment of heroin addiction can be found.

This hope, however, is based on a misunderstanding. One main advantage of methadone is that it *is* addicting. For an addicting drug, it will be recalled, is one that an addict continues to take day after day and year after year.

In fact, several nonaddicting drugs for the treatment of heroin addiction have already been tried out. Among them

[2] From *Licit and Illicit Drugs: The Consumers Union Report on Narcotics, Stimulants, Depressants, Inhalants, Hallucinogens, and Marijuana, Including Caffeine, Nicotine and Alcohol,* by Edward M. Brecher and the Editors of *Consumer Reports.* Little. '72. p 159-62. Copyright © 1972 by Consumers Union of United States, Inc. Reprinted by permission of Little, Brown and Co.

are the narcotic antagonists; cyclazocine and naloxone are examples. An addict who injects heroin while on one of these drugs perceives no effect. Thus the antagonists, like methadone, are "blocking agents." But they are inferior to methadone in at least two other major respects.

First, they do not assuage the postaddiction syndrome—the anxiety, depression, and craving that recur for months and perhaps years after the last shot of heroin. The contrast with methadone is readily visible. A psychiatrist who has had experience with both methadone and antagonist maintenance programs contrasts "the relaxed, jovial atmosphere of a methadone ward," where patients are free of the postaddiction syndrome, with "the tension, frustration, and anxiety that characterize a cyclazocine ward." [*Science*, 173:505. August 6, 1971] Clearly methadone is in this respect a far more hopeful base for building social rehabilitation.

The other major difference is that since the antagonists are not addicting, a patient can stop taking them at will. (Dr. William R. Martin, chairman of the Addiction Research Center at Lexington, and the scientist who first proposed use of narcotic antagonists in the treatment of heroin addiction, reported (1971): "Patients learned that by skipping doses they could experience the euphorogenic action of [taking] heroin the day following the last dose of cyclazocine." [*New York Law Journal*, 166:34. December 6, 1971]) Most patients do stop taking them—and then promptly return to black-market heroin. The greater success of methadone results in considerable part from the fact that it is an addicting drug.

In 1971, despite the earlier failures of narcotic antagonists, interest was renewed in these drugs as a potential "cure for addiction." (The most recent study of cyclazocine, reported in the *International Journal of the Addictions* [John N. Chappel, Edward C. Senay, and Jerome H. Jaffe, "Cyclazocine in a Multi-Modality Treatment Program: Comparative Results," *International Journal of the Addictions*, 6:509–523. September, 1971] in 1971, indicates that of 186 addicts offered cyclazocine, 33 accepted, of whom 11 were believed to be abstinent twenty months later. The study suggests, but does not prove, that the few patients who accept cyclazocine do significantly better than similar patients who attempt abstinence without cyclazocine.) A massive research program was proposed for an improved antagonist, or for an improved way of administering those currently available. It was suggested, for example, that a long-term supply or "depot" of an antagonist might be implanted somewhere in the addict's body, surrounded by a membrane that would release the drug at the desired rate continuously over a period of a month or even six months. If such a long-acting material were available, it was argued, addicts could be *required* to take it at suitable intervals, under penalty of imprisonment. Hence, it was said, such a drug might solve the addiction problem, even if addicts didn't like the drug.

What the large-scale use of a long-acting narcotic antagonist would in fact produce, however, is a horde of men, women, and adolescents assailed by anxiety and depression, with a continuing craving for heroin—and no way to assuage their distress (except, perhaps, via alcoholism). Is this the "cure" society seeks for today's narcotics addicts? (The civil-liberties implications of requiring the taking of a drug that not only perpetuates anxiety, depression, and craving but also blocks relief of that syndrome for prolonged periods deserves fuller consideration than was given the subject during the 1971 discussions of long-acting narcotics antagonists.

(An ethical consideration is also involved in the use of long-acting narcotic antagonists: why is it *wrong* to provide an addict with an addicting drug such as methadone—that is, one that carries a built-in pharmacological compulsion for continued use—but *right* to use legal compulsion, even imprisonment, to force continued use of a nonaddicting drug?)

Despite the shortcomings of the narcotic antagonists as a "cure for addiction," further research into these drugs could prove valuable. For the central facts of addiction—

the withdrawal syndrome followed by the postaddiction syndrome—are still little understood. The study of narcotic antagonists is quite likely to throw further light on the mystery of why some drugs merely block the heroin effect while others—notably methadone—both block the heroin effect and relieve the depression, anxiety, and craving for heroin.

It is unfortunate, of course, that patients must continue to take methadone year after year, just as it is unfortunate that diabetics must continue to take insulin or some other diabetes drug year after year. But the heroin addict's need for continuing medication is *not* the result of methadone; it arises out of his initial addiction to heroin. Methadone relieves the patient of the life-shattering effects of that need.

A patient on methadone maintenance is commonly thought to be addicted to methadone and might therefore be called a methadone addict. (Dr. Marie Nyswander disputes this common view. She points out that a methadone maintenance patient who discontinues methadone does not develop a craving for methadone and does not go looking for methadone. Instead, his craving for *heroin* returns and he goes looking for heroin. Hence, he is not, in common parlance, addicted to methadone. He is an ex-heroin addict who is relieved of his heroin addiction so long as he takes his methadone. [Marie E. Nyswander, personal communication]) The term "methadone addict" is seriously misleading, however, since—as we have seen—the patient on methadone maintenance does not resemble in the least the popular stereotype of the addict. He neither acts like an addict nor thinks of himself as an addict. To avoid confusion, the terms *heroin addict* and *methadone patient* have become standard usage, and are used throughout this Report.

If being legal and being cheap were methadone's only advantages, one would expect methadone maintenance to be neither better nor worse than morphine maintenance or heroin maintenance. But in four other significant respects, methadone is distinctly superior to either morphine or heroin as a maintenance drug. The first of these advantages is that methadone is fully effective when taken by mouth. [Vincent P. Dole, "Thoughts on Narcotics Addiction," *Bulletin, New York Academy of Medicine*, 41:212. February, 1965] Thus the whole long, tragic list of infections spread by injection needles is eliminated at one fell swoop. Infections due to morphine and heroin injection can be minimized by dispensing them in sterile ampules with nonreusable needles, but the oral drug is obviously a further improvement.

Second, methadone is a *long-acting* drug. An adequate oral dose in the morning keeps the user on a relatively even keel until the next morning. (An even longer-acting drug related to methadone—acetyl-alpha-methadol—is said to be effective for three days or longer and may ultimately replace methadone as a maintenance drug. [See Vincent P. Dole. "Thoughts on Narcotics Addiction."]) Stabilized methadone patients do not "bounce" from "sick" (incipient withdrawal symptoms) to "nodding" (excessively tranquilized). Addicts on morphine or heroin, in contrast, must "shoot up" several times a day, and many of them bounce.

Third, some addicts, as noted above, have a tendency to escalate their doses of morphine or heroin. Once stabilized on an adequate daily dose of methadone, in contrast, patients are content to remain in that dose year after year; [Vincent P. Dole and Marie E. Nyswander, "Rehabilitation of Heroin Addicts after Blockade with Methadone," *New York State Journal of Medicine* p. 2015. August 1, 1966] some even ask to have the dose reduced. Thus the main problem of morphine and heroin maintenance programs— the dosage problem—is readily resolved.

Methadone's fourth advantage is that it *blocks* the heroin effect. [Vincent P. Dole and Marie E. Nyswander, "Narcotic Blockade—A Medical Technique for Stopping Heroin Use by Addicts," *Transactions of Association of American Physicians,* 79 (1966):132] A patient stabilized on an adequate daily dose of methadone who shoots heroin discovers to his own amazement that it has no effect—that he has wasted his money. The higher the methadone maintenance dose, the larger a dose of heroin is thus blocked. The methadone dose can be set at whatever level is necessary to block the largest heroin dose a patient is likely to secure. (In Britain, where large doses of unadulterated medicinal heroin are available, much larger doses of methadone are dispensed than in the United States—up to 400 milligrams per day, for example, as compared with the usual 100 milligrams daily here. [Personal communication]) There is nothing mysterious about this blocking effect; it is just a special case of cross-tolerance. Any opiate or synthetic narcotic, in a given dose, will block the effects of any other opiate or synthetic narcotic given in a substantially smaller dose. The Dole-Nyswander program merely makes use of this well-known relationship among opiate and synthetic narcotics to discourage the use of heroin while on methadone.

No "high" or "bang" or "rush" is experienced when methadone is taken by mouth in regular daily doses. Indeed, nothing whatever is experienced except the taste of the orange drink in which methadone is dissolved. To demonstrate this, Drs. Dole and Nyswander occasionally gave patients who came in for their daily dose of methadone a placebo instead. The patients couldn't tell the difference. Not until hours later, when withdrawal symptoms began to appear, did they realize that they had not received methadone. When methadone is mainlined, however, some people get much the same reaction that some people get from heroin. This is one reason why methadone for maintenance use is dispensed in a hard-to-inject, soft-drink or tablet form in the United States. In Britain, physicians are permitted to prescribe—and some do—injectable methadone for addicts.

Finally, methadone staves off not only the acute effects of withdrawal from heroin—a fact long known—but the postaddiction syndrome of anxiety, depression, and craving as well, year after year. On methadone the patient no longer thinks constantly about heroin, or dreams of it, or shapes his whole life to ensure a continuing supply. He no longer engages compulsively in "drug-seeking behavior." He is, quite soon after going on methadone, freed of the heroin incubus. In this sense, he is "cured."

These advantages of methadone, however, should not be interpreted as criticisms of legalized heroin or morphine maintenance, as practiced in Britain today and in Kentucky earlier, for example. While the latter are no doubt inferior to methadone maintenance in the respects described above, they are still a vast improvement over the American heroin black market.

NARCOTICS: ANOTHER TREATMENT [3]

The Bristol-Myers Company has developed a new type of methadone which it says will reduce illegal traffic in the drug as well as other abuses.

Announcement of the new drug coincided with the disclosure by Dr. Dominick J. DiMaio, . . . [New York City's] acting medical examiner, that the methadone now in use killed almost twice as many people here last year as heroin did.

DiMaio said 181 deaths were caused by methadone poisoning in 1973 compared to 98 attributable to heroin. He said a full report would be released . . . [soon].

Dr. Irwin J. Pachter, research director for Bristol Laboratories, said the new drug—called Methanex—contains the "narcotic antagonist naloxone" which, when taken orally, works like ordinary methadone but, when injected, causes the user

to experience the pains of withdrawal—as if he had suddenly kicked the habit "cold turkey." Because of this effect and the fact that methadone and naloxone are virtually impossible to separate, the new product will reduce the temptation to divert methadone from treatment centers to the black market.

[3] Newspaper article in the New York *Post*. p 10. Ag. 16, '74. Reprinted by permission of New York *Post*, © 1974, New York Post Corporation.

He explained that Methanex comes in three forms: a bulk powder, an effervescent tablet and a non-water-soluble tablet.

The first two forms have been approved by the Federal Drug Administration, Pachter said, and "will be offered to treatment centers and clinics throughout the nation immediately." The non-water-soluble tablet, he said, has been approved for sale to selected centers on an experimental basis pending further study.

This tablet has the further advantage of lending itself to color-coding so that, if it does show up on the black market, it would be easy to identify "treatment centers which are sources of diversion" he said.

Dr. Robert Newman, director of methadone maintenance programs for [New York City's] Health Services Administration, said his department was "going to investigate it and see if it does have advantages for us, but at the present we have no plans to convert to Methanex."

TWELVE SUGGESTED STEPS
OF ALCOHOLICS ANONYMOUS [4]

1. We admitted we were powerless over alcohol—that our lives had become unmanageable.

2. Came to believe that a Power greater than ourselves could restore us to sanity.

3. Made a decision to turn our will and our lives over to the care of God *as we understood Him*.

4. Made a searching and fearless moral inventory of ourselves.

5. Admitted to God, to ourselves and to another human being the exact nature of our wrongs.

6. Were entirely ready to have God remove all these defects of character.

[4] Excerpt from *Young People and A.A.*, pamphlet published by A.A. World Services Inc. '69. p 38. Copyright © 1969. Reprinted with permission of A.A. World Services, Inc., copyright owners, P.O. Box 459, Grand Central Station, New York, N.Y. 10017.

7. Humbly asked Him to remove our shortcomings.

8. Made a list of all persons we had harmed, and became willing to make amends to them all.

9. Made direct amends to such people wherever possible, except when to do so would injure them or others.

10. Continued to take personal inventory and when we were wrong, promptly admitted it.

11. Sought through prayer and meditation to improve our conscious contact with God, *as we understood Him,* praying only for knowledge of His will for us and the power to carry that out.

12. Having had a spiritual awakening as the result of these steps, we tried to carry this message to alcoholics, and to practice these principles in all our affairs.

DRUGS AND THE YOUTH SUBCULTURE [5]

The Haight-Ashbury: Its Predecessors and Its Satellites

During the 1960s, young people in substantial numbers —most of them middle-class and white—migrated to the Haight-Ashbury district in San Francisco. Adopting strange hair and clothing styles, they rejected the platitudes of their parents and of the "square" communities from which they came, coining unconventional platitudes of their own. The mass media called them *hippies*. A major feature of the hippie life-style was the use of illicit drugs—many different illicit drugs.

Nothing quite like this, it was commonly believed, had ever happened before—but that belief was mistaken. The "youth drug scene" of the 1960s was a continuation, under a new name and with minor changes in external style, of a continuing social process. Even in external appearance, the hippies of the 1960s—and the beatniks of a decade earlier—

[5] From *Licit and Illicit Drugs: The Consumers Union Report on Narcotics, Stimulants, Inhalants, Hallucinogens, and Marijuana, Including Caffeine, Nicotine and Alcohol,* by Edward M. Brecher and the Editors of *Consumer Reports.* Little. '72. p 491-507. Copyright © 1972 by Consumers Union of United States, Inc. Reprinted by permission of Little, Brown and Co.

markedly resembled the "bohemians" who made their first appearance in Paris in the 1840s, founding a movement that spread to the United States. Male bohemians, like male hippies, let their hair grow long; they and their female counterparts dressed in a manner deemed uncouth by the bourgeoisie. Bohemians lived in poverty in attics resembling today's hippie "pads." They held unconventional philosophies and flaunted unorthodox sexual mores.

The Timothy Leary of the bohemian movement was Henri Murger (1822-1861), a Parisian whose *Scènes de la Vie de Bohème* (1848) established and popularized the bohemian life-style; but Murger's greatest influence, and the peak popularity of bohemianism, came after 1898—when Puccini's opera *La Bohème*, based on Murger's *Scènes*, achieved worldwide renown.

Like today's hippies, the turn-of-the-century bohemians were conspicuously drug-oriented. One of the drugs that the bohemians (like their elders) used was alcohol. Murger himself became an alcoholic at an early age, and died in a sanitarium at the age of thirty-nine. In addition to alcohol, the bohemians used coffee. They drank vast quantities of this stimulant, were preoccupied with coffee, and suffered coffee as well as alcohol hangovers. Respectable citizens of that era were as horrified by the bohemian coffee cult as today's respectable citizens are horrified by marijuana smoking. Eminent scientists, it will be recalled, echoed this horror; for it was at the height of the bohemian coffee cult that the public [in 1909], was being warned: "The sufferer [from coffee addiction] is tremulous and loses his self-command; he is subject to fits of agitation and depression. He loses color and has a haggard appearance. . . . As with other such agents, a renewed dose of the poison gives temporary relief, but at the cost of future misery." [Sir T. Clifford Allbutt and Humphrey Davy Rolleston, eds., *A System of Medicine*, vol. II, part I, pp. 286-287. London, Macmillan, 1909]

The Haight-Ashbury of the 1960s also resembled New York City's Greenwich Village of the 1920s, another center to which rebellious young people migrated. In the Greenwich Village era, it was the short, "boyish-bobbed" hair of the girls (rather than the long hair of the boys) along with their miniskirts, lipstick, and breastless "John Held, Jr." silhouettes, that shocked society. Necking, petting, and nonmarital sexual adventures were widely publicized features of the Greenwich Village scene and life-style.

The Greenwich Village subculture of the 1920s featured two drugs. One of them was alcohol. During the Prohibition years, socially rebellious young people from all over the United States thronged Greenwich Village's illicit "speakeasies" to drink "bootleg" liquor. The fact that young *women* were getting drunk in public, and could be seen staggering out of speakeasies at all hours (for a part of the cost of Prohibition was an end to the enforcement of legal closing hours) added to the popular revulsion.

The other Greenwich Village drug habit that deeply outraged the respectable was cigarette smoking. In 1921, it will be recalled, cigarettes were illegal in fourteen states and 92 anticigarette bills were pending in twenty-eight states. Smoking cigarettes in speakeasies and other public places was almost as alarming to some respectable members of society as engaging in nonmarital sexual encounters. Young women (Edna St. Vincent Millay among them) were expelled from college for smoking cigarettes much as in the 1960s young women were expelled for smoking marijuana.

In each generation, moreover, the drug-subculture phenomenon was not limited to the bohemian quarter of Paris, to Greenwich Village in New York, or to Haight-Ashbury in San Francisco. "Little Bohemias," patterned on Murger's Parisian original, could be found all over the Western world —including American cities from New York to California. Similarly, bush-league Greenwich Villages sprang up throughout the country during the 1920s, and bush-league Haight-Ashburys followed in the 1960s. These deviant youth cultures, characterized by bizarre clothing, unconventional hair styles, sexual nonconformity, and illicit or "bad" drug use, were not only national but international. London, Stockholm, Copenhagen, Amsterdam, Rotterdam, Montreal, Vancouver—all have hippie neighborhoods.

Finally, each of these life-styles also attracted "internal migrants," who patterned themselves on the deviant youth-drug-cult style of life without actually leaving home. Retired schoolteachers now in their seventies can no doubt remember the early 1920s, when almost every high school, even in Iowa and Kansas, had its "Greenwich Village crowd"—drinking bootleg alcohol, smoking cigarettes, "necking," "petting," reading the *American Mercury,* and writing poetry, to the distress of respectable citizens. Today, many (perhaps most) high schools have their pot-smoking, acid-dropping deviant youth subcultures composed of "internal migrants" who stay at home. In what follows, references to "youth-drug-scene migrants" will include these internal migrants.

What happened to rebellious young people in between these luridly publicized waves of youth-culture migration and internal migration? While the available evidence is sparse, it suggests that essentially the same process continued, on a smaller scale, with less flamboyance and less popular alarm. Every large city in the nineteenth and early twentieth century had its crowded, rundown "rooming-house district," sheltering not only its alcoholics, brothels, and streetwalkers but also youthful migrants in large numbers. Young artists, young writers, and young musicians— along with even larger numbers of would-be artists, writers, and musicians—flocked to these "Skid Rows," "Tenderloins," and "red-light districts." While prostitution was generally limited to such neighborhoods, only rarely were the red-light districts limited to prostitution. Low rents and the sense of freedom and adventure attracted countless youhful migrants to the same areas. Many eminent Americans, such as Stephen Crane, Theodore Dreiser, and Ben Hecht, participated in this scene. The drugs in most common use were usually alcohol and nicotine—though youthful deviants at times (as noted above) also turned to opium smoking and to cocaine, morphine, heroin, or a combination of such drugs.

The use here of the term *deviant* should not be deemed a value judgment; it is a purely descriptive term. In any generation, a majority of young people tend to follow the path marked out for them by the society in which they find themselves. A minority deviate from this path. One group, for example, drops out of junior high school; another group continues through graduate school. Both groups, in this context, are *deviants* from the usual path.

During the nineteenth and early twentieth century, sermons, newspapers, and sensational popular fiction were the chief media informing young people of the perils of bohemias and of rooming-house and red-light districts—and incidentally publicizing their precise locations. The movies added their influence during the Greenwich Village era. The TV screen, the popular musicians and singers, and the mass media *en masse* played a generally similar role in publicizing the youth drug scene during the 1960s—and with similar results. It is hard to say whether romantic glorifications of such scenes or moralistic warnings against their perils contribute more to attracting rebellious young people to them.

In all eras, law enforcement has also played a crucial role in publicizing Greenwich Villages and Haight-Ashburys. The periodic nineteenth century "vice squad" crackdowns on rooming-house and red-light districts, the Prohibition agents' raids on speakeasies during the 1920s, and the multitudinous drug raids by narcotics agents during the 1960s —each wave of raids accompanied by a wave of sensational publicity, and by pictures of young people defiantly confronting the police—added to the glamor of the youth cult centers, and made it certain that even the naivest teenager in the remotest country village knew (and currently knows) precisely where to go and approximately how to behave, including what drugs to try, when he or she reaches the scene.

Against this briefly sketched historical background . . . the current youth drug scene can perhaps be more objectively understood and evaluated.

One potentially fruitful way to view the youth drug scene today, like the bohemias, rooming-house districts, and Greenwich Villages of earlier generations, is as a *competing* way of life. Such scenes compete with conventional institutions and life-styles for the allegiance of each youthful generation. The more young people find unattractive the way of life mandated by their elders at any moment in time, the more they are likely to run off, or wander off, or embark on an internal migration toward what appear to be greener pastures.

A curious fact about deviant youth subcultures must next be noted. *In each generation, respectable society itself dictates the direction that much of the deviance will take.* During alcohol Prohibition, for example, hostility was focused on alcohol—and it was alcohol that rebellious young people drank. Through the 1960s, society dictated *drug* deviance to young people, and that was the path youthful deviants followed.

This concept of *dictated deviance* can best be understood through a prototype example. Consider the anxious parents who keep watch over their unmarried teenage daughter for fear the daughter will become pregnant out of wedlock. The parents harp on dire warnings of the perils of illicit intercourse, accompanied by emotion-laden accusations and predictions: "Where were you all evening? Whom were you out with? Why weren't you home on time? You're going to get yourself pregnant and ruin your life and ours—we can see it all coming."

The daughter gets the message loud and clear: "If you want to get even with your parents (or with society in general) for grievances real or imagined, the best way is to get yourself pregnant." The peril becomes a lure, and the prophecy proves self-fulfilling. In almost precisely this way, society as a whole dictated drug use as the dominant mode of deviance for disaffected young people during the 1960s. "Watch your step. Be careful. We can see it all coming. You're going to start smoking marijuana and progress to heroin. You're going to end up a hippie!"

No doubt a few years in a nineteenth century bohemia or in Greenwich Village in the 1920s contributed positively to the maturing of many young people of those generations. Certainly a number of distinguished writers, artists, musicians, even philosophers, came through such deviant youth scenes. Whether the same will prove true of contemporary Haight-Ashburys remains to be seen.

There can be little doubt, however, that future histories of music will cite the youth drug scene of the 1960s as one of the transforming influences on musical development. Whether psychedelic art will similarly survive seems less certain. Future histories of religious mysticism may well hail the current Haight-Ashburys as the sites of a major religious resurgence comparable to New England transcendentalism in the days of Emerson and Thoreau. Canada's Le Dain Commission in particular has stressed this possibility:

We have been profoundly impressed by the natural and unaffected manner in which drug users have responded to the question of religious significance. They are not embarrassed by the mention of God. Indeed, as Paul Goodman has observed, their reactions are in interesting contrast to those of the "God is dead" theologian. It may be an exaggeration to say that we are witnessing the manifestations of a genuine religious revival, but there does appear to be a definite revival of interest in the religious or spiritual attitude towards life. As one drug user put it: "The whole culture is saying, 'Where is God?' I don't believe in your institutions, but now I know it's there someplace." Another witness said, "I just find that a lot of people are becoming a lot more aware of what's happening and joining in on a universal cause, a cosmic sort of joyousness and people are getting interested in spiritual things as well, because this is what our generation and the previous generations have lacked. . . ." [*Le Dain Commission Interim Report*, pp. 157-158]

Society's evaluation of today's Haight-Ashburys may ultimately be raised, as the accepted evaluation of the Greenwich Villages of the 1920s has already been raised. For now, many view the youth drug scene as an unmitigated evil and want to know what can be done about it. Three suggestions arise out of the above analysis.

First, a good way to lessen the likelihood that young people will migrate to the youth drug scene, or to any other form of social deviance, is to make the conventional pattern of life back home more attractive and challenging to young people—better able to compete with the deviant alternatives.

Second, a good way to decrease the likelihood that young people will select the youth drug scene rather than some other mode of deviance is to turn off the propaganda and the warnings that center so much attention on drugs—and thereby in effect dictate *drug* deviance.

Third, the number of participants in the youth drug scene at any moment depends only in part on how many young people enter it; the other determining factor is how many graduate from it and how soon they graduate. Thus one way to curb the Haight-Ashburys, large and small, is to keep the door wide open so that drug users can emerge from the scene. . . .

Why a Youth Drug Scene?

If the view is accepted, at least tentatively, that each generation spawns a larger or smaller proportion of deviant young people, and that these young people through the decades have sought for and found a deviant scene and lifestyle, complete with their own costume, hair style, drugs, and sexual mores, a further question arises: why do *drugs* play so central a role in the currently dominant pattern of deviance?

The data are not yet available for a definitive answer. But a few factors are already clearly visible. The first concerns, not the deviant scene itself, but one's perception of it.

Throughout the past century, society has tended to focus its dismay on two areas of youthful behavior—drugs and sex—and to condemn deviance from generally accepted standards in either area. In recent years, while still on occasion deploring sexual nonconformity, society appears to be much more concerned with illicit drug use among deviant subcultures.

Again, young people discovered during the 1960s that the conventional drug sequence prescribed by society—from caffeine and nicotine to alcohol—is not an inexorable law of nature. . . . Many young people had excellent reasons for seeking alternatives to alcohol. The use of other drugs by some young people in the 1960s can thus be viewed as a well-intentioned effort to escape the evils of alcohol.

LSD and marijuana were the first alternatives to alcohol to be widely publicized. Once freedom of choice and black markets were established, however, the spectrum broadened enormously. Young people, white and middle-class, began to experiment with a wide variety of different drugs—including, after about 1969, heroin. Unfortunately, that concept of choice and that experimentation arose at precisely the time when this country's antidrug propaganda was furthest out of touch with reality and therefore least credible.

To sum up, national drug policy throughout the 1960s contributed to the rise of the current youth drug scene in at least four major ways. First, by emphasizing "drug abuse," it virtually dictated youthful *drug* deviance rather than other forms of deviance. Second, by publicizing marijuana, LSD and LSD-like drugs, the amphetamines and other stimulants, the barbiturates and other depressants, and the opiates as well, these pronouncements informed an entire generation of the broad range of mind-affecting drugs from which a choice could be made. Third, for many the warnings actually served as lures. And finally, the supposed facts provided to inform and guide young people turned loose in the contemporary illicit-drug supermarket were almost invariably incredible, in conflict with everyday experience. Hence young people were left to flounder along without guidance they could trust—to learn by their own trials and errors and those of their peers.

The errors young drug users made, of course, were numerous—and some of them were tragic. This we all now know. But the extent to which well-meant, sincere, but disastrous antidrug policies contributed to the tragedies is still only vaguely perceived, or not perceived at all.

First Steps Toward a Solution: Innovative Approaches by Indigenous Institutions

Young people have many problems, whether or not they use drugs. They get sick and need medical care. They get toothaches and need a dentist. They get in trouble and need a lawyer. They get lonesome and need friends, plus a place to meet with their friends. They need food and a place to sleep. They get confused and need wise counseling. In addition, if they use drugs imprudently, their problems may become more complex.

The first waves of youthful migrants to Haight-Ashbury in San Francisco, to the East Village of New York City, and to the other youth drug scenes during the 1960s brought with them their full share of such problems, and acquired new ones in the drug scene. To help them with these problems, indigenous institutions arose—centers that were themselves a part of the drug scene, and that were established to meet the needs of drug-scene participants rather than the needs of the "square" society outside. Some of the institutions were staffed by ex-drug users (some of whom might still smoke marijuana on occasion); others were founded by sensitive adults who recognized hippies as human beings with many human needs.

The indigenous service agencies set up to help drug users are so numerous and so varied as almost to defy description. We shall here describe, accordingly, only a few significant prototypes. We shall consider them at some length and with great seriousness, however; for out of these youth-oriented service centers there are currently emerging both the first reliable insights into the nature of the deviant youth drug subculture and the most hopeful approaches toward solving the manifold problems of illicit drug use. In contrast to high-sounding policy formulations at the national level, the drug scene's indigenous institutions are evolving policies out of their day-by-day confrontation with the practical problems of today's young people, including but not limited to their problems with drugs. When effective approaches to this country's "drug crisis" are ultimately adopted, they will almost certainly include solutions currently being pioneered by these informal, loosely organized, and apparently haphazard local institutions within the drug scene itself.

"Switchboards" and "hot lines." During San Francisco's 1967 "Summer of Love," when adolescent "flower people" descended upon the city from all over the United States, a young resident of the Haight-Ashbury named Al Rinker realized that there was an urgent need for a primitive communication system—a place where young migrants could get answers to pressing questions:

"I'm sick; how do I get to a doctor?"

"I'm broke. Where can I get a pad for tonight? A hot meal? A bath?"

"I'm pregnant; now what do I do?"

"My girl friend has just slashed her wrists. Help!"

Parents, too, needed a communications center:

"Where can I find my daughter? She's fifteen, has red hair, and wears lavender-tinted glasses."

"Can you find my son and tell him his mother died last night?"

In an effort to meet such needs, young Rinker publicized his personal telephone number in the underground press and elsewhere; calls promptly came pouring in. Volunteers, some of them drug users, helped him man the phone around the clock. Friends contributed small sums of money. Additional phone lines were installed. The service moved to larger quarters in the Haight-Ashbury. Thus arose one of the first and most urgently needed of the indigenous drug-scene institutions, the San Francisco Switchboard. Similar "hot lines" were soon in operation in other drug centers. To-day there are several hundred hot lines, at a rough estimate, operating in towns as small as twenty thousand, as well as in most large cities. The best of them are concerned not only with drug problems but with the countless other problems young people today confront.

"Rap centers" and "crash pads." Alcohol drinkers have countless places to meet, talk, and drink—saloons, taverns, cocktail lounges, roadhouses, and night clubs, to mention only a few. The first migrants to the youth drug scenes had only their overcrowded pads and the streets. Help soon came, however, from a limited number of broad-minded churches, neighborhood centers, libraries, and other helping agencies, which set up "rap centers" where young people could meet, talk, rest, listen to music, escape from the streets. Some rap centers took the form of coffeehouses, others adopted other patterns. Many, not all, have rules against using illicit drugs on the premises; all or nearly all have rules against dealing in illicit drugs on the premises. (A number of cities in the United States and other countries have also tolerated places—sometimes called "coffeehouses" —where young drug users can congregate and smoke mari-juana; but these are not subsidized public agencies. "Turn-ing on" has been similarly tolerated at some rock-music festivals and other large-scale youth gatherings. The city of Amsterdam in the Netherlands has gone considerably fur-ther; it has made available public buildings and subsidies from tax funds for "rap centers" and music centers (such as the widely publicized Paradiso) where marijuana and hash-ish are publicly smoked. Many visitors to Amsterdam are amazed by this tolerance. One explanation is that city of-ficials want to keep young people off the streets; another possible motive may be a desire to strengthen the marijuana-hashish culture at the expense of the opiate culture, the am-phetamine culture, perhaps even the alcohol culture. Per-

haps, too, Amsterdam's city fathers genuinely want to help meet the needs of young people as they try to meet the needs of other segments of the population. The fact that Amsterdam's young people have their own political party and elect their own representatives to the city council is probably also relevant. It is possible that the recent lowering of the voting age to eighteen here in the United States may have similar results.)

"Crash pads"—that is, rooms with cots or at least mattresses where young migrants can spend a night or two— have similarly sprung up within the drug scene, in association with hot lines and rap centers or independently, sponsored by churches and other helping institutions or founded by drug users themselves. The rap centers and crash pads may be staffed by concerned volunteers, or they may boast a paid (minimally paid) staff of "indigenous nonprofessionals."

The useful functions of these centers are numerous. For one thing, they serve as news centers where young people can find out what is going on. (The scene is rarely the same from one season to another; new drugs, new ways of using and misusing them, and new nondrug problems are constantly turning up.) The centers also disseminate important information—such as warnings against a fresh shipment of worthless drugs, or of especially damaging drugs. Again, these centers are the places where peer standards are generated and peer pressures applied. The pot smoker who stays stoned all day, for example, or the "head" who drops acid too often, or the "speed freak" who shoots too much amphetamine over too long a period, or who engages in other forms of self-defeating, group-endangering behavior, can here be called to account by his fellow drug users.

Such peer pressures within the drug scene are far more effective than official or educational warnings. They do not, it is true, work miracles. They do not convert a compulsive drug user into a total abstainer. But neither does the conventional warning: "If you take LSD, you'll end up in a mental hospital." The goal of the rap centers, crash pads, and other indigenous drug-scene institutions is to *minimize the damage* done to young people by drugs and by other adverse influences. This goal, however modest, has at least the merit of being achievable.

The need for meeting places for young people was set forth in a speech by Canada's Minister of Health John Munro before the British Columbia Medical Association on October 5, 1970:

> Most of all, drop-in centers—drug-free, harassment-free spots where young people can come around to mix and talk with people whom they consider their brothers and sisters—are an absolute must. Many people feel that their development should go hand in hand with the erection of the proposed national hosteling network. [John Munro, in *Canadian Medical Association Journal*, 103:1100. November 7, 1970]

This Munro speech, quoted further below, is particularly important because it demonstrates how a wholly new approach to the problem of illicit drugs, replacing traditional methods of repression, can be made *politically* palatable to voters. The *Canadian Medical Association Journal*, which called it "one of the most forceful and understanding speeches of [Munro's] political career," reprinted it at length in its November 7, 1970, issue.

"Crisis intervention centers." Young drug users, like other human beings, young and old, face crises from time to time. A crisis may be drug-related—an LSD "bad trip," for example, or a "crash" following a prolonged "speed run." Or a crisis may be simple exhaustion due to sleeplessness and malnutrition rather than drugs. Again, the presenting symptom may be mental depression, drug-associated or not; such depressions can reach suicidal intensity among young people as well as older people, among abstainers as well as drug users.

Such crises outside the drug scene are ordinarily handled by the emergency rooms of local hospitals; and before the rise of the indigenous drug-scene institutions we are describing, participants in the youth drug scene also tried the hospital emergency rooms. They also sought help at first from established clinics, welfare agencies, social work organizations, and other helping institutions. With some notable exceptions, however, these agencies proved poorly adapted to the needs of youth-drug-scene participants.

Many established agencies tended to view the crisis as essentially a *drug* problem, and sought to solve it by persuading the young patient or client to abstain from drugs altogether. Young drug users responded by walking out and staying away.

Many established agencies at first disapproved of the hippies' hair style, costume, sex mores, and style of life generally —and did not hesitate to make their disapproval known. Young long-hairs responded by staying away.

Many hospital emergency rooms and other established agencies asked questions and adhered to rules and regulations. Many refused to serve minors, for example, without written parental consent. Proof of local residence was also often required. Many participants in the youth drug scene were both minors and migrants; they responded to the questions and regulations by simply staying away.

Many established agencies felt called upon (as required by some state laws) to report drug users to the police. Once such police reports were made, the grapevine spread the news—and young drug users stayed away.

The youthful drug user who went to an indigenous "crisis intervention center" instead of to a hospital emergency room met with very different treatment. This was *his* place, set up to serve *his* interests. No questions were asked. The staffs of the indigenous centers, moreover, gradually learned from day-to-day experience improved methods of handling crises. In hospitals, for example, LSD "bad trips" or "freakouts" and other LSD emergencies were generally treated in the early days by administering tranquilizers and other medication. The staffs of the crisis intervention centers learned instead to "talk a man down," using reassurance, friendliness, diversion of attention, and other simple psychological methods to calm the panic. Only the most serious cases required a physician, or hospitalization. Unlike the hospitals, the crisis intervention centers did not simply turn patients loose after the crisis was over, or call the police. Postcrisis counseling was available—at the moment when it was most likely to be effective.

"Free clinics." Just as Al Rinker founded the original San Francisco Switchboard on his own initiative, so Dr. Joel Fort founded the first "free clinic" in San Francisco in 1966; and Dr. David E. Smith and a few physician associates, acting as volunteers, founded the Haight-Ashbury Medical Clinic during San Francisco's 1967 "Summer of Love," to meet the medical needs of the youth drug scene migrants. Currently an estimated fifty to eighty other "free clinics," modeled more or less closely on the Fort and Haight-Ashbury patterns, are functioning in major drug centers from coast to coast. Some are subsidized by voluntary contributions, others also receive funds from local health departments. These clinics are "free" in the sense that no charge, or only a nominal charge, is made for services. The term "free" also indicates, however, a clinic free of the traditional rules, regulations, and attitudes.

The following 1970 prospectus for a Montreal "youth clinic" illustrates the principles common to most free clinics:

As you may be aware, there exists today a large population of youth who are not seeking the advice and help of established medical facilities for their problems. These problems include . . . normal difficulties found in that population, as well as specific disorders related to the nonmedical use of drugs and to sexual activity, e.g. drug-induced mental disturbances, unwarranted pregnancies, venereal diseases, etc.

One approach to the problems mentioned above has been the establishment of "Youth Clinics," organized and directed by the youth population, and located in a community center setting, which patients do not regard as foreign or hostile. 4424 Youth Clinic is such an establishment and is now in operation. It is permanently staffed by a physician and a psychiatric social worker. Clinics are held in general medicine, gynecology and psychiatry.

Additional staff work on a voluntary basis and include residents from the Queen Elizabeth and Montreal Children's Hospital as well as volunteers from the youth center. A full range of medical services is provided; referrals to specialists in the out-patients' departments are made when necessary. There is no fee for service and medications are provided free of charge if the patient is unable to pay. One of the major factors in the success of this type of clinic is that complete confidence between patient and doctor is maintained: parents are not informed without the knowledge of the patient.

The aim of the clinic is threefold:
1. Treatment
2. Prevention
3. Crisis Intervention

Typical illnesses treated include mouth and chest infections, skin diseases, allergies, venereal infections, etc. as well as psychiatric problems of adolescence and disturbances related to drug use.

Prevention includes the following:
1. Information on drug hazards given in a factual and nondogmatic manner, i.e. the most recent scientific data concerning drug hazards
   (a) dangerous drugs currently being sold in the street
   (b) procedure in case of bad drug reaction
2. Information on venereal disease and birth control
3. Drug information to parents and the community at large, thus narrowing the "generation gap" aspect which motivates many youths to risk taking dangerous drugs to defy their "straight" parents

Crisis Intervention will include a twenty-four-hour telephone service where a doctor can be reached to treat a bad drug reaction, as treatment in hospital emergency wards are not only often inadequate but may even be detrimental. [*Interim Report for 4424, Inc.,* Youth Centre/Clinic, Montreal (1970); unpublished]

By common consent, anyone coming to a free clinic for help is deemed to be eighteen years of age—or whatever age is locally required for treatment without parental consent. There are no local residency requirements. No unnecessary questions are asked. The police are not informed. If requested, only the patient's nickname is recorded. Even the shabby psychedelic décor of the clinic is designed to make participants in the youth drug scene feel welcome and at home. The physicians staffing the free clinics are mostly

young volunteers who give their spare time or else are minimally paid; few have short haircuts or other stigmata of
respectability.

Canada's Health Minister John Munro vividly described
these free clinics, known in Canada as *street clinics,* in his
1970 address:

Perhaps the best answer is one which blends in emergency
drug care with the rest of the spectrum of medical practice. I refer
to the street clinic. After all, many illnesses crop up among drug
users which are only indirectly related to the drugs they take.
They come more from the dropout life-style of the heavy user,
which is itinerant and mendicant. They include malnutrition
from a diet rendered insufficient either by personal poverty or by
the type of drug used. They also include the full gamut of respira-
tory ailments, from coughs and flu to chronic bronchitis and
pneumonia, stemming from overexposure to inclement weather in
inadequate clothing, and compounded by nutritional deficiencies.
They also include VD. They include hepatitis and other varieties
of vascular infection resulting from dirty needles.

To deal with this constant demand for basic health care, the
street clinic locates itself in the neighborhood of its primary clientele. As a matter of fact, its staff members may more closely
resemble the clientele than they do regular health personnel. As
in one case we ran into recently, the central doctor may have
shoulder-length hair, and wear a headband and serape. So located and staffed, the clinic takes care of medical problems of all
varieties, not just crises. And it doesn't require documentary
proof of Medicare coverage before extending treatment. [Medi-
care in Canada covers all ages.] Thus it is more than a clinic;
it is a refuge for those who are not welcome at numerous regular sources of care, or mistrust them, or want at all costs to avoid
the identification procedures which are followed there.

Thus, these centres are vital, and I hope that they will spread.
I also hope that their development is plotted hand-in-hand with
municipal and regional health planning agencies, so that the
clinics have the necessary back-up for major cases, which may lie
beyond the scope of their own capacity. [John Munro, in *Canadian Medical Association Journal,* 103:1097]

The quality of the medical care delivered by these free
clinics is not always high; *but it gets delivered.* In the process, it subtly affects the attitudes and behavior of youth

drug scene participants. A warning against a new drug shipment which has just hit town, for example, achieves an altogether different credibility rating if it comes from a free
clinic rather than from a traditional agency—for several
reasons: First, the free clinic does not destroy its own credibility by issuing unrealistic warnings. Second, the free clinic
has earned respect as a truly helping agency; its warnings
are therefore perceived as designed to serve the best interests
of drug users themselves rather than repressive goals. Third,
the free clinic's advice is based on its own experience. It can
therefore be readily confirmed by a drug user's personal observations within the scene. Much the same is true of warnings circulated by other institutions indigenous to the drug
scene; but because of its medical orientation, the free clinic
is the most authentic source of reliable drug information,
and is perceived as such by its patients.

Most medical problems handled by the free clinics are
not drug-related at all. Indeed, when asked what service
drug users need most urgently, clinic physicians often cite
dental care.

As the free clinics and other indigenous institutions have
established their usefulness and earned respect from both
the "square" and the "hip" communities, they have been
increasingly successful in bridging the chasm between drug
users and established institutions. The clinics have accom-
plished this in part by interpreting the drug users to the
established hospitals, clinics, welfare and other agencies, and
in part by interpreting the established institutions to the
drug users. As a result, patients and clients requiring medical or other services beyond the scope of the free clinics are
now being referred to established institutions with much
less of a "hassle," and with greater likelihood of a favorable
outcome. Where drug users feel they are being treated un-
fairly, the free clinic can sometimes intervene effectively in
their behalf.

Comprehensive drug-scene centers. The newest, rarest,
and most hopeful development among the drug scene's in-

digenous institutions is the appearance of a few *comprehensive* centers combining all of the functions described above, from hot line and rap center to free clinic—and offering in addition a wide range of other services including education and prevention. In particular, these comprehensive centers are concerned with two as yet unanswered questions:

How can emergence from the youth drug scene be encouraged and facilitated?

How can the recruitment of additional participants be discouraged? . . .

Are these indigenous institutions, from hot lines to comprehensive youth centers, worthy of public support—even though their primary goal is to help drug users rather than to repress drug use? Canada's Minister of Health John Munro eloquently stated the case for generous support in his 1970 speech:

After all, it is our children we are talking about. And some of the drug users of today will be the leaders of tomorrow. Will they come to power with a fierce dedication to destroy everything we now represent—the good along with the bad—because of the way we now treat the drug problem? Or is there still time to show them the "system" is flexible enough to understand them, help them, and accommodate their valid opinions about the necessity of social change? [John Munro, in *Canadian Medical Association Journal,* 103:1102]

WELCOME TO THE CLUB [6]

The courtroom of a suburban community, normally a quiet place, was filled one day recently with a large group of high school and college boys and their parents. The boys were being arraigned on charges of possessing or selling marijuana, LSD, barbiturates, and amphetamines. They had been rounded up early that morning from their homes by

[6] "Welcome to the Club: An Attitude," Chapter 9 from *Children and Their Parents,* by Suzanne Strait Fremon. Harper. '68. p 153-76. Copyright © 1968 by Suzanne Strait Fremon. Reprinted by permission of Harper & Row, Publishers, Inc. Mrs. Fremon is a frequent contributor to *Parents' Magazine* and other periodicals.

officers of the police narcotics squad, brought to the police station to be booked, and were now being called up to the bar by name, one by one, and informed of the charges against them, and asked whether they were guilty or not guilty. Every one of them answered, "Guilty."

Their faces were closed down. One boy, in fact, covered his face with his hands the entire time he was in the courtroom, until the judge required him to drop his hands and raise his head. Several others hid their faces whenever they had to turn toward the audience or the newspaper photographers. But some of the boys revealed their feelings in other ways: several swaggered noticeably when they were called up; one boy bit his fingernails savagely. Another, whose mother tried to put her arm across his shoulders, jerked himself away from her.

The parents, well dressed and obviously middle-class suburban Americans, had clearly been taken by surprise. Some were stunned. One mother wept. One father muttered to himself. Another kept trying to break into the proceedings to talk about his rights. They carefully avoided each other's eyes.

One woman said in a high, carrying voice, "I'm in shock. He was never deprived of anything. Do you know what this does to us? We'll have to move."

A father said, apparently to himself, "I can't believe it. I can't believe it. I can't believe it."

The district attorney pointed out to newspaper reporters that all the boys were in good high schools or colleges, came from families who lived in expensive houses or apartments, and owned at least one car and more often two. He said, "These are not dropouts, or slum kids, or disadvantaged kids. As a parent, I feel great compassion for the parents of these youngsters. This is undoubtedly the most tragic day of their lives."

He was probably right. A generalization about these boys and their parents is risky, of course, but no matter what the background of each family situation and the degree of involvement in lawbreaking of each boy, for any parent in such a situation this is a bleak day. Their responses are as varied as their natures: anger at the authorities, anger at their sons, self-castigation, disbelief, surrender, grief, elaborate rationalizations. And the feelings on which the responses are based are just as varied: anxiety, love, hostility, pride, concern, fear, uncertainty, bewilderment, disappointment, even indifference. Buried deep in each parent's memories, and lending another dimension to the scene in the courtroom, are the scenes from other years: the little boy, the baby, the twelve-year-old, the neighborhood gang, the school assembly, the Cub pack—years of pictures. And the feelings these pictures evoke, the memories of other feelings: pride, amusement, love, and above all, the dreams.

What happened to the boy in those early pictures? And where did the pride give way to worry or bewilderment? And when did the dreams disappear? And the cry of anguish: *what's the matter with these kids anyway?*

Every parent of nearly grown children knows some of these feelings. Where, oh, where did the children vanish? The adorable, curly-haired, three-year-old boy, the sturdy Little League pitcher, the timid little girl, the pigtailed tomboy: vanished. And in their places are large people with deep voices and opinions and private lives of their own. It is a bittersweet experience at best for parents to watch their children become adults. Yet the parents of young people who are growing up well can at least see, if they pause and look back, how each came to be the way he is now. A large part of the tragedy of the parents in the courtroom is that they do not know how their sons came to be there. What were the steps? Someone made some mistakes: who? when? what mistakes? And the corollary of this tragedy is another: not understanding the causes in the first place—or the boys, either—they have no idea how to help their sons now, or themselves, or how to prevent it from happening again with these same boys or with others.

Those of us whose children are apparently not caught

up in the use of drugs are frightened when we read of the scene in the courtroom. Any parent of adolescent children whose head is not buried in the sand must be aware that he knows very little of what goes on in his children's lives. There but for the grace of God—or luck, or good management, or what?—go our children. And the question mark in that sentence is the most significant part of it.

We are frightened, first of all, of course, for those specific boys. They appear to be engaged in an activity that is both illegal and personally harmful. They come from families whose members customarily support the law, and the attitudes and customs from which the laws are derived. Lawbreaking, then, represents a long step away from their background, in an unknown direction. In addition, drug taking is a dangerous occupation, and these boys are not so stupid nor so ignorant that they do not know this fact and recognize at least some of its implications. An additional observation: these kids are dissatisfied with their lives—with their parents, their schools, the United States Government, and with mankind in general.

From this view of these few boys, parents immediately turn their attention to the whole generation. What's the matter with all these kids? Why do any of them take drugs? And here we stick: most of us know next to nothing about drugs. And we begin to suspect, with a terrible falling of the heart, that we know next to nothing about our children. Children and drugs: a new problem, with no identification with anything in our own lives. Perhaps this is where we must part company with our children's generation. Perhaps we are doomed not to understand it.

On the other hand, if we compare drug taking, which we know very little about, with drinking, which most of us, from experience and observation, know a great deal about, we may shed a little light on the question. Why do people drink too much? We all know there are dozens of answers to that one. One man drinks too much because he has a messy marriage—and one of the reasons for the messy marriage is that he drinks too much—and he would rather be lightly drunk than entirely sober when he is at home. Another has a job he hates but cannot leave, and he sees the days of his life departing forever in boredom and frustration and disappointment. Another thinks he is a writer but somehow cannot seem to write much of anything. Another drinks because he likes the sexual results. Another because life just looks better through an alcoholic haze. Still another drinks because his friends do and he likes the parties every Saturday night. Another just drifted into it and over the course of a dozen years has established a firm habit. And so on.

The boys in the courtroom are too young to have the same piled-up intensity of feeling behind what drug taking they are actually engaged in, but they may have many of the same basic reasons: problems they cannot solve and yet cannot abandon; a dismal personal future; the wish to get along with friends; habit; lack of anything better to do; and to top it all off, a view of the world that is too depressing to take straight.

In addition they have the problem of their own independence. Any experienced parent knows that a spirited child of any age goes to enormous trouble to establish his independence from his parents. The specific episodes vary greatly, according to the temperament of the child, as well as his age and stage of development, but from his first "No!"— whether spoken or gestured or expressed in an angry wail— he asserts himself, his own self, over and over again through the years against the will of his parents. During high school years in particular children are engaged in separating themselves from their parents. In fact, sometimes they seem to be doing little else. And the taking of drugs, or at least the appearance of drug taking, provides a current group of young people with an effective way of achieving and displaying independence.

We must remember one more thing as we look at the sad little group of boys in the courtroom: from here we cannot tell at all which of them has been pushing drugs all winter among his high school friends in a most cynical and destructive way and which ones were simply experimenting for the first time with the experience. For that reason we cannot even begin to answer the question, "Why did they do it?" because first we must ask, "What exactly did they do?"

They did something illegal: that is about all we can say for sure. And no reasonable adult human being would maintain that all illegal activities are equally serious. The courts recognize this, of course; many schools do, too, to their credit. Newspapers are less likely to; and local gossip circles are least likely of all to differentiate between the boy who has been introducing illegal and dangerous drugs into his school and pushing them hard among young and ignorant kids and the boy who is cautiously experimenting with a marijuana cigarette for the first time. The moment their names are published, or even known around town whether or not they are printed in the papers, all the people involved are assumed to have been equally guilty of equally serious offenses.

This is not to defend the use of marijuana among high school and college students. Enough defenders are already speaking out: marijuana is no more addictive than cigarettes, they say; it is certainly no worse than alcohol; and look at the use of tobacco and alcohol among adults—it's phony and hypocritical of them to object to a little marijuana. The fact is that, although cigarettes may not be addictive in the strict medical sense, any smoker who has ever tried to give up smoking knows from the inside the terrible force of that particular habit. And to say that marijuana is not worse than alcohol is to say also that it can be very bad indeed. Almost everyone over the age of forty has seen what twenty years of drinking do to some human beings: among other things, alcoholism. A sizable group of twenty-year-old college students at a drinking party probably contains at least one future alcoholic: can anyone in the group identify him? Of course not; and least of all the future alcoholic himself. "It can't happen to me." Besides, the age of forty is so far in the future that no sensible twenty-year-old is concerned with it. Nevertheless, all adults know that middle age eventually arrives and brings with it the full-grown versions of the problems that were planted twenty years before. Marijuana is not as immediately destructive as LSD; just the same it has its own dangers, and twenty years of drug taking, of even a relatively "harmless" drug, can bring problems that no one in his senses would deliberately cultivate. Finally, to say that adults should not preach about drugs because look how much worse they are themselves is to be childish in one's attitude and illogical in one's thinking. "Do as I say, not as I do" is not the most persuasive argument in the world; nevertheless, most parents really want their children to be better than they are, not worse. And a father who has blown half a dozen big chances in his life because he got drunk at the wrong time may want more than anything to help his son avoid that particular trap.

At the same time that we reflect on all this we must recognize that the high school and college students who try marijuana to see what it does to them are not necessarily headed straight for the narcotics ward. Again, there are parallels with the use of alcohol and tobacco: most of the parents and grandparents of these boys and girls experimented in exactly this way with drinking, or smoking, or both. Some of them tried it and abandoned it; some tried it, liked it, and stuck with it in moderation; some tried it, got hooked, and spent years of their lives alternately battling it and succumbing to it; some are killing themselves with it; and some are already dead from it. The same opportunities are open to our children in their smoking and drinking and their use of drugs.

The question then arises: how can we help our own children to find their way through this forest of opportunities? Clearly, we cannot protect adolescent children from exposure to drugs, and most sensible parents would not if they could. But neither can we leave them entirely without guidance in a matter that will affect them as long as they live and may even have a bearing on the time and the manner of their death.

As parents, perhaps the most difficult problem we have is to see the situation—any situation, not only the questions posed by drugs—in the context of a child's whole life and the whole climate he lives in. We tend to respond to a specific episode as though it stood alone and had no causes leading up to it and no results leading away. The mother in the courtroom who said, "I'm in shock. He was never deprived of anything. Do you know what this does to us? We'll have to move." This mother is obviously blind to the influences that brought her son to this room, and her first thought of the consequences of the situation has to do with the need to move to a place where no one will know about it. She has no view at all of her son as he really is: a solitary human being standing at the intersection of two lines of force: a horizontal line representing his immediate surrounding—his family, his school, his interests and activities outside of school, his friends—and a vertical line representing the span of his life, from infancy to old age. She thinks some muddled version of "Look what he has done to us! What can we do to him so he won't do it again? Or so people won't know if he does do it again?"

Unfortunately for our children's sake, it is easier to condemn this mother than it is to find constructive attitudes and practices for ourselves. When we look at a child, one of our own children, and at a situation he is in, thinking about these two lines of force that act on him, trying to understand what he needs, what the specific situation really is, what the background is, and what the future probably holds, we may find ourselves in a muddle, too, so much so that we cannot say or do anything at all helpful to him. And yet we must. And so we blunder along, saying the things that seem to us to be most important and a lot of irrelevancies besides, giving the warnings and pointing out the hidden pitfalls, often unnecessarily, describing some of the possible benefits, often of dubious value to the young, and in general doing our poor best, hoping it is adequate.

In such a muddle as this parents can sometimes find the most sturdy guidance for themselves, and indirectly for their children, in general principles distilled from their own attitudes and temperaments, and preferably expressed in a form that is oversimplified for quick reference in an emergency. A conversation with almost any parent of children who have grown successfully from childhood to adulthood will reveal a handful of these principles that he has developed through the years and that continue to guide him in his dealings with children. A mother says, "I always say 'Yes' unless there is an important reason for saying 'No.' " A father says, "You have to be absolutely truthful with your kids all the time, even when it seems unimportant. Otherwise how can they possibly trust you when they need the truth?" Another mother: "I always try to be at home from three o'clock on every day." Another father: "I always try to explain things to him the best I can." These are all expressions of attitudes that have guided these adults in their relationships with their children, and like all such expressions, each of them is the small visible part of a large submerged body of belief that determines the general climate of family life. The mother who tries to say "Yes" is clearly an accepting, trusting woman who believes in the capacities of her children to cope with whatever "Yes" will bring to them. The father who makes a point of telling the truth has plainly thought out the implications of not telling the truth. The mother who stays at home when her children may need her understands the importance of the physical presence of parents and the father who takes the trouble to explain understands the importance of teaching his children what he himself has learned. Each of these parents presents to his children an integrated point of view, a solid base upon which to build a relationship, and a consistency that will support that relationship.

Another attitude that is demonstrably successful can be

expressed by saying, in effect: "Welcome to the club; here are the rules." This, too, is an oversimplification, of course, but a family that operates with this kind of attitude as a base is not likely to have to go to court to hear one of its members plead guilty to charges connected with the illegal use or sale of drugs. In an earlier chapter the suggestion was made that perhaps the most valuable single quality in a growing child, and the most important one to help him develop, is self-confidence. In the same spirit, this chapter suggests that the most helpful attitude of parents toward their growing-up children may be this one: Welcome to the club.

We welcome our children into the world. Most parents are delighted when their children are born. We send word to all the kin everywhere and to friends across the country: this child is born. We do this much before we can say anything at all about him beyond his sex and his weight. Even so, we are delighted. We are thrilled when he starts school and enters the world of formal learning that will make available to him the experience of all mankind that has gone before him. We welcome him into various organizations as he grows—churches, scout troops, museums, libraries, teams—and we make special efforts to teach him how to be a good member of each one. But many of us fail to welcome our children into the biggest and most important organization of all: the adult world.

Our failure may be due partly to our own defensiveness. When the young attack the old, the old feel for the first time the clammy breath of their own passing. We see that we are being threatened by time, in the persons of our own children. A man may be forty-five, a scratch golfer, and one of the leaders of his corner of the world, with twenty years of increasing productiveness ahead of him, but when his twenty-year-old son gazes at him coolly and smiles in the superior twenty-year-old way, the father may feel the cold all the way to the marrow of his bones. And instead of seeing his son as a bright boy with great eagerness to learn and glorious visions for the future, he sees him as a callow stripling with no experience and boundless intolerance. Actually the boy is all these things: bright, callow, eager, inexperienced, intolerant, visionary. The father chooses the qualities he will see, and his choice is dictated by his own fears. Instead of teaching his son, then, and helping him gain the experience he so sadly lacks, and encouraging him to follow his visions, the father tends to rebuff him; or distrust him; or belittle him; or antagonize him. In short, instead of smiling and saying, "Welcome to the club," this father is shaking his head and saying, "You don't qualify for membership."

To look upon the whole of the adult world as a club may strike many adults as taking an impossibly cozy view. The world is an unattractive place in many of its aspects. At its worst it is hideous. Even at its best it is a complex beyond understanding of all but a handful of its inhabitants. To admit this and then in the same breath maintain that it is a club is perhaps even to be irresponsible.

Yet by thinking of ourselves as a gigantic club we can protect ourselves to some extent from the despair that might swallow us up if we insisted on standing alone against the hideousness and complexities. All of us who are living through our lives at the same time on this planet are of necessity concerned with the same problems, and we are all trying to do the best we can with what we've got. This is justification enough for forming a club, electing officers, adopting a constitution and a set of bylaws, and holding a meeting now and then to hear from each other. In addition, we do need some mechanism for taking in new members to run the club as the old members die.

Children are not yet full voting members. In time, however, they will be, whether we like it or not, and conscientious parents spend the days of their lives preparing their children for responsible, productive membership. And if the job is well done, the children will assume their membership gradually, bit by bit, as they slowly acquire an understanding of the world and of themselves, and of the way they will fit into the world and the world will fit around them. They do not suddenly "grow up," obviously. They develop slowly with spurts and setbacks, depending on their own natures and on the accidents of their lives, over a period of many years, until imperceptibly they turn into adults.

His parents are often the last people to realize that a child is grown up. They have been scrutinizing the boy too closely for too many years to be able to see the whole man when he appears. Frequently, this recognition is ludicrously delayed. One father, for example, learned it suddenly after a family Thanksgiving gathering, when his son came for the day with his wife and two small children. The young man, with no idea that his father was suddenly seeing him with new eyes, treated the older man as usual, with affection and respect, disagreed calmly with him half a dozen times, and went off at the end of the day with his own young family to his own house, unshaken, serene, able to cope with his world. His parents looked at each other with discovery in their eyes: this child was finally an adult. He was a member of the club.

He had been an adult for some time, of course. And although his parents had not seen this quite so clearly or so soon as his wife saw it, or his boss, or his friends, they had been encouraging his growth since he was born, and instead of being dismayed they were overjoyed when he finally began to act all of a piece, as a grown-up member of the human race. . . .

The second half of the expression of this attitude is: "Here are the rules." All clubs have rules by which members govern themselves. The adult world has many such sets—laws, customs, manners, and many more informal but accepted ways of acting and reacting—and although they vary greatly from country to country, and although they overlap and sometimes even come into conflict with each other, the general principle holds wherever we look: every group with even a rudimentary organization has rules. Even the groups of young people that appear to most adults to be most anarchistic have their own accepted ways of acting and dressing and being. In fact, a group of hippies in New York who run an apartment where apparently anyone who needs a place to sleep can find a place and a welcome have a rule that is considerably more stringent than the rules that govern most places: no drinking, no drugs, no minor girls.

Any serious effort to train children for membership in the world of adults, then, must include an effort to describe to them as fully as possible the reasons for those rules. This is a lifetime job, carried on by many agencies all the time, and it is not always successful. But one of the best ways a family can help in this larger operation is to establish a set of rules for family life.

This is not to say that the only reason for family rules—or even the main reason for them—is to train children to understand and accept the rules of society. From a sociological point of view a strong family organization helps all of society to be strong and from a psychological point of view a strong family organization helps the individuals to be strong. But even if these things were not true, families would still have rules to govern their own family life because family life would be chaos if they did not.

Naturally, every family's rules are individual and they differ, sometimes markedly, from those of other families. They reflect an enormously complex background—the individual social and economic history of each of the parents, the immediate social circumstances of the family, its income, the personal preferences of the members, their temperaments, and their relationships among themselves. But no matter how they have arrived at their rules, every stable family finds itself developing over the years a set of patterns ranging from the most general attitudes by which the members deal with each other to specific regulations to take care of money, social engagements, and household responsibilities, down to who washes the dishes on Saturday nights.

Whatever the differences in detail or even in general expectations that exist among families, one general statement appears to be true: successful families base their family life, whether or not they are aware of it, on a feeling of confidence in each other. That is, the adults trust each other and trust the children; the children trust each other and trust their parents. This means that all the members of such a family have confidence in all the others to act from decent motives, to try to avoid hurting each other, to tell the truth, and to contribute in some reasonable way to the general welfare of the family. . . .

The members of this family expect each other to behave well. And as a result of those expectations they do behave well. The children in such a household will not be defensive, because their parents will not forever be looking for infractions of the rules. . . . The parents in such a family will be not defensive either. Their authority is not at stake every time they make a suggestion; they will come to see themselves as senior members and officers of the club—or teachers, or guides, or in whatever role fits their concept of the group—rather than as dictators ruling over inferior beings. And the family atmosphere in general is pleasant: it consists of confidence, mutual assistance, affection, and a genuine pleasure in each other's company.

This atmosphere of confidence comes under the greatest strain, probably, when children begin to grow up and turn their backs on the family and begin to take on the coloration of some other group. Some young adolescent children appear to arrive at this point while they are still physically at home and going to high school. Many more wait until they are in college or away at school or at work. The parents are hard put to believe that the child who arrives in the house for Christmas vacation with his hair four inches longer than it used to be—could it possibly have grown that much since September?—and wearing sandals in spite of the cold and dark glasses in spite of the pouring rain is the same boy who graduated with honors from the local high school last June, complete with sunny smile, scrubbed face, and several awards from the faculty. And the boy sees his parents in a new light, too. They have not actually changed: they still get up early in the morning and go about their lives with their friends and their jobs, watching television, going to meetings, or parties, or golf games as they have always done, but he suddenly sees this life as stifling and hideously wasteful. In fact, both parties to the relationship are no different from before but they see each other differently. And this weakens the bonds of trust that existed for so long. Can this kooky kid really be expected to get through college, looking the way he does, and, good Lord, when you think what it costs! And can these stodgy parents really be relied upon to understand what I want to do with my life, living the way they do? Both parents and children doubt it. Uncertainty creeps in. Caution enters. Hostility pokes a head around the door. Defensiveness springs up. And conversations, which used to be pleasant and productive, are now tense and unsatisfying, and perhaps cease altogether. Neither side quite trusts the other. And the club, which was a pleasant association of human beings of different ages and talents, all pursuing the same general goals, suddenly becomes an enforced confederation of enemies. Once the hostility is allowed to take over the atmosphere, all the years of trust are in jeopardy. No longer do the members expect each other to behave well. The parents, having characterized their son as "kooky," expect him to behave like a kook. The son, having characterized his parents as stodgy and dull—worse, as hypocrites and phonies—then sees everything they do as additional proof of these qualities.

Parents put in the hardest work of their lives as parents trying to avoid this situation and not all of them—not even the ones who try hardest—succeed. It would be much easier, and perhaps just as effective, if they could kiss their children *au revoir* at the age of eighteen, or even sooner with some children, and commit them to the part-time care of someone else until they arrived at adulthood, whenever that finally came. All the basic parental work has been done long since, certainly. Whatever judgment the child is going to bring to his problems is already at work in his character. He can certainly find advice every bit as good as he is likely to get at home almost anywhere he goes. And any honest adult knows that at times a family is as much an emotional burden as it is a help. This arrangement would remove most of the pain from the relationship between nearly-adult children and their parents.

Unfortunately, it would also remove much of the pleasure. With the exception of those women who honestly prefer tiny babies to any other form of human life, most successful parents tend to like their children and enjoy them more with every passing year. Beginning at the age of about four months, when a baby stops being undifferentiated Baby and shows the faint beginnings of what he will eventually turn into, he improves steadily as a member of the family and as a companion. By the time he is in his teens he can be a joy, a source of interest and pride, and a fine addition to family gatherings. This can be the most rewarding period of all for his parents. It would be a pity to miss it simply to save the pain of having to get along with the thorny creature.

This is where a specific family rule can come into play: keep each other informed. In the polysyllabic world of the social sciences this rule comes under the heading of "communications," and a family that ignores it or in some other way fails to achieve it is commonly said to be suffering from a breakdown in communications. What they are really doing, of course, is simply not talking to one another. This can be a dangerous situation: a family whose members are ignorant of one another's thinking and feelings and doings is operating far below the level of effectiveness it might achieve.

Keeping one another informed involves an amount of talking and listening and thinking and responding that frightens some people: it covers so much territory, they say, and it takes so much time. And so it does. The information that members of a family convey to one another in the course of keeping informed ranges from the most specific and trivial to the most general and important. "We're going to the pizza place." "Jeff's party will be over by 11:30." "We've been held up; be home in an hour." "I got a C– on the test." "Listen to this story, it's funny." "The saddest thing happened today." "It was so beautiful I cried." "She cheated." "I got so mad I punched him." "He doesn't understand." "You don't understand." "I don't understand." "If you'll leave me alone, I think I can manage." "I don't know whether to take physics or not." "Billy says he's in love with me." And so on and on.

It is only by means of this kind of reporting, through years of telling each other what is on their minds that two people can ever come to know each other well and to understand each other. But a mother and a daughter who talk steadily to each other for twelve years probably know each other well enough by the time the girl is fourteen so that nothing she does will surprise her mother and whatever responses the mother has will seem reasonable to the girl. "Oh, mother wouldn't like that." "How do you know? Did she ever tell you not to?" "No, but I know she wouldn't." And a girl of fourteen whose mother has listened to her carefully and sympathetically and then has responded carefully and honestly for twelve years is much influenced by what she thinks her mother would or would not approve.

Boys appear to talk to their parents less than girls. The various myths that govern the growing up of the male versus that of the female—and some of them may be based on real differences, who knows?—may tend to inhibit open discussion by many boys of their feelings and thoughts. This is a pity, because this reluctance to discuss attitudes and feelings often results in a reluctance even to think about these things. And this, in turn, results in some stunting of their understanding of themselves. And the whole situation can eventually come to a point where an adolescent boy and his parents have almost nothing to say to each other.

This kind of situation arises in almost every household at one time or another, probably. The great hulking adolescent boy slumps in front of the television set hour after hour watching professional football while his mother flits nervously in the background, wondering and worrying. Or the college girl home on vacation closes her door firmly against her parents and spends her whole time in the house lying on her bed writing long letters to unknown correspondents, or listening to the radio and dreaming, while her mother hovers outside the door, wanting to talk to her but not wanting to be rebuffed.

Some of this is inevitable. But some of it must come from rebuffs in the other direction. Even the most relaxed and friendly parents have occasions when they cannot treat their children in a relaxed or friendly way. We are human beings, too, as we all know, with problems of our own, and these problems often need attention that causes us to look away from our children and fail to hear them when they speak. We cannot expect our children to pay any attention to these, but we must also accept a standard lower than the highest possible level if we want to try to keep on trying.

In addition, the changes that are taking place in society put a strain on family conversations. Every parent of adolescent children has surely had the experience of hearing a sentence from the child that went straight to the solar plexus and knocked the wind out of him. At a moment like this a parent who wants to keep the conversation going will call on reserves he had no idea he possessed and will maintain the same facial expression, the same tone of voice, and even more important, the same confidence in the child, at the same time that his mind is reeling and he is saying desperately to himself, "Dear God, what have we here?" This is a lot to expect from a mother whose nineteen-year-old daughter has just announced as she scrubbed a kitchen pot that her major problem at the moment is whether or not to go to bed with Joe. But if the mother wants to be of use to her daughter at all in this important area she had better listen and not cut off the conversation with a horrified comment, or a sermon, or even a lecture designed to show how

enlightened she is. Even if she suspects her daughter is show-
ing off a little, or testing the water to determine the temperature, she had better take the whole matter with the
degree of seriousness it deserves and respond to it with every
bit of honesty and helpfulness she has in her. She must
proceed on the assumption that her daughter wants to talk
about it or she would not have brought it up; even more,
the daughter may actually want to listen. Perhaps she really
wants to know what her mother thinks and feels and believes.

In her efforts to be honest the mother must sooner or
later express her real reaction to her daughter's dilemma,
whatever that reaction is. And here, often, is a large block.
Either the mother is unalterably opposed to her daughter
sleeping with Joe, for a combination of reasons she can
hardly put into words, or she is very nearly as confused as
the daughter as to the rights and wrongs of such a step. Almost never would she say, either in words or in manner,
"Go right ahead, dear. Hop into bed with him if you feel
like it." And either of the paths she feels like following—
definitely opposed to it or honestly not having a clear-cut
opinion about the principles involved—has its own dangers
for the conversation. In such a situation she might remember that if the daughter herself were sure she would have
hopped long since, and the girl honestly wants some kind
of conversation about it. Also, in addition to her disadvan-
tages as a consultant, the mother has one overriding advantage: she is not in love with Joe, and as a result her view
of what is right and wrong is likely to be more reliable than
her daughter's view.

Many mothers of present-day adolescent boys and girls
find the whole idea of discussing one's sex life over the dinner dishes repellent in the extreme, and this attitude tends
to stand in the way of honest dialogue, too. They would
never initiate it themselves. On the other hand, dinner
dishes, like driving and riding in a car, provide something
to do with one's hands and eyes, which helps when it is

necessary to use words and phrases that many middle-aged women have seldom said aloud. Also, a mother in such a situation might reflect that she did not initiate it and it is not her sex life that is under discussion: it is her daughter's, and her daughter presumably does not mind.

This is a dramatic example of the kinds of pitfalls that await a family where the members try to keep each other informed. It is far from being the only kind. From their child's earliest years, when a little boy filches a cherished toy from a friend in kindergarten and suffers until he confesses to his mother and returns it, to the day when he comes home from college and says he wants to drop out, and even beyond, parents who are willing to listen to their children are faced with the consequences of their willingness: they will be told things that will trouble them, keep them awake nights, call into question many cherished notions, and once in a while shake them up so that they will never be the same again. On the other side of the coin of this distress, however, will be the dawning realization that almost nothing they hear will be the end of a story; they will be brought into most episodes early in the action, at a point where they may be able to influence it a little, and certainly at a stage where their understanding and whatever wisdom they can muster up will help the children. The five-year-old boy who stole the toy is no thief, any more than the nineteen-year-old girl is a tramp, or the college boy a bum. They are all troubled people who need help from somewhere. If they can find it at home, the chances are extremely good that they will never become thieves, tramps, or bums.

When a family adopts the attitude of "Welcome to the club," and when they say, in addition, "Here are the rules," they are also implying one more statement. This is: "Any suggestions?" A well-run club has a mechanism for changing the rules; a wise management adopts an attitude that when the members want the rules changed they are at liberty to try to change them. The members of the club who are in control at any moment—the Establishment, so to speak—are

willing to listen to the newcomers. This attitude implies
open-mindedness to new ideas, a readiness to change. It does
not mean that whatever the new members want they should
automatically have simply because they are young and energetic and filled with ideas. Their parents were once young
and energetic and filled with ideas, and they have learned
that while some of these ideas were good ones and worked
well when they were tried out, some of them were terrible,
and life might have been easier if there had been someone
around to say, "I tried that back in nought-eight and fell
flat on my face." The least we can do for our children is to
say to them, "I tried that back in thirty-eight and fell flat on
my face." Sixty-eight is a different world, granted, but so
was thirty-eight, of course. The question "Any suggestions?"
means that we will listen—really listen—to suggestions, and
then use our best collective judgment to decide whether or
not the suggestions are good.

This attitude can be developed and displayed from the
time the children are very young. "That's not fair!" This is
one of the eternal cries of childhood. And sometimes the
child is right; it is not fair. And sometimes the parent is the
one who is being unfair. Here the child is bringing an acute,
uncorrupted sense of justice to a situation and lodging a
complaint with the club management. What will the club
management do about it? Turn away, saying, "It's one of
the rules; no appeal"? Or, "Oh? Isn't it fair? What's unfair
about it?" And then after listening—really listening—be
willing to explain in full why it really is the fairest thing
under the circumstances or to change the ruling to make it
more fair.

Unfortunately, there are several groups of growing children who are highly resistant to the attitude of "Welcome
to the club." Some of these are the children who are naturally silent, born loners. These people simply decline to keep
other people informed about themselves and are apparently
genuinely indifferent to information about other people.
These people make poor members of any club, although

most of them eventually seem to join something, if only to establish families of their own. They may lead active inner lives, and frequently they are among the most interesting and productive human beings of their generation. But in their growing-up years they can cause anguish to their parents, who cannot tell, often, whether a boy is simply being silent or turning surly, or whether he is in control of his life or in such a turmoil that he cannot express it. In their adult years these people seem to continue to be more interested in their own inner lives than in any aspect of the outer world. "He's all right, I guess," says the mother of one such boy. "But I can't really tell. He doesn't tell me enough so I can judge. I suppose he's all right." This kind of comment may represent a situation that is acceptable, even interesting, to a growing boy; to his mother it is a source of pain and worry, and finally resignation. The chief real difficulty in the lives of these children is that when they genuinely need help of some kind they may not know how to go about finding it: they are not accustomed to expressing themselves to other people; they are not accustomed to asking for help; they are not accustomed to accepting help. They give themselves serious trouble that they might have avoided on account of their inability or unwillingness to express themselves somehow. It is worth trying long and hard to establish some kind of channel so that a boy or girl of this kind can see a way of reaching help when he needs it.

There are other children to whom membership in any club of which their parents are members is highly distasteful. Some of these youngsters may show up in groups of rebels of various sorts, establishing themselves in clubs of their own with different sets of rules. They choose occupations as far removed as possible from their parents' occupations. They distrust the motives of everyone of their parents' generation or even the generation halfway between them and their parents. This attitude is hard on their parents, of course, but from an objective point of view, or from the point of view of the youngsters themselves, it may be sound and productive. Very few parents can achieve this kind of objectivity about their own children: a child who leaves home in rebellion and sets himself up as far from home as possible in a way that is clearly a rejection of home and parents, and who scorns his parents and everything they stand for, is attacking his parents in such a direct way that they cannot be expected to be patient and understanding about the situation or the child. But from the point of view of the world as a whole this kind of reaction may be healthy and sane. The youngster may be acting instinctively from a sense of self-protection, or even from a sense of survival. He is fleeing from a place he does not like, and from people who apparently do not want him as he is, to a place where he is comfortable and to people who say to him, "Welcome."

These young people are certainly better off than those tragic figures who have come to be known as "alienated youth." These poor children are rejecting not only their parents but the whole world. They find their reality—or what passes for reality with them—in the fantasy world of drug-induced hallucinations. Beside these sad creatures a bearded, sandaled, campus activist preaching on behalf of peace on earth is a young man to cherish and support. His parents may remember the peace marches of their own generation—some of them on the eve of World War II, of course—and conclude that such actions are but candles in the wind. But these parents must also reflect that mankind's deep desire for peace must find expression in every generation and if the expression brings beards and sandals along, too, what of it? These young people are involved in the real issues of the real world and they are unlikely to give it up for a pretend world of drugs.

Most children, in fact, want eventually some kind of fully accredited membership in the adult world. This does not mean that they accept the world as it is, any of them. Even the most compliant would change some aspects of it if he could, and it is a safe bet that every single adolescent is compiling an informal list in the back of his head of things

his parents do that he will never, never do. And while they yearn to be adults, these almost-adults have moments of self-doubt and fear of the adult world, and many of them put off joining it as long as they can, but they all overcome their fears sooner or later. Each of them comes to see that the world is the only one there is and the life he is living is the only one he has to live in the world, and he had better get at it.

Surely the most helpful attitude a parent can take as his child is working his way slowly toward this decision is one of welcome. "Welcome to the club. Here's the way we run it. Any suggestions?"

BIBLIOGRAPHY

An asterisk (*) preceding a reference indicates that the article or part of it has been reprinted in this book.

BOOKS, PAMPHLETS, AND DOCUMENTS

*Alcoholics Anonymous. Rose joined A.A. at 16. A.A. General Service Office. 468 Park Ave. S. New York 10016. '69.
*Alcoholics Anonymous. Twelve suggested steps of Alcoholics Anonymous. A.A. General Service Office. 468 Park Ave. S. New York 10016. '69.
Alfonsi, Philippe and Pesnot, Patrick. Satan's needle: a true story of drug addiction & cure. Morrow. '72.
Andrews, Matthew. Parents' guide to drugs. Doubleday. '72.
Anslinger, H. J. and Tompkins, W. F. Traffic in narcotics. Funk & Wagnalls. '53.
Austin, B. L. Sad nun at Synanon. Pocket Books. '71.
*Ausubel, D. P. Drug addiction: physiological, psychological, and sociological aspects. Random House. '58.
Baden, William. The private sea: LSD and the search for God. Quadrangle. '67.
Barber, T. X. ed. Drug abuse and drug education. Random House. '73.
Barnette, H. H. Drug crisis and the church. Westminster. '71.
Baudelaire, C. P. Artificial paradise: on hashish and wine as means of expanding individuality; tr. by Ellen Fox. Herder & Herder. '71.
Bell, R. G. Escape from addiction. McGraw. '70.
Blakeslee, A. L. Alcoholism—a sickness that can be beaten. (Public Affairs Pamphlet no 118A) Public Affairs Committee. 381 Park Ave. S. New York 10016. '74.
Blum, R. H. and associates. Society and drugs: social and cultural observations. Jossey-Bass. '69.
Blum, R. H. and associates. Students and drugs: college and high school observations. Jossey-Bass. '69.
Blum, R. H. and others. The dream sellers: perspectives on drug dealers. Jossey-Bass. '72.
Blum, R. H. and others. Drug dealers—taking action: options for international response. Jossey-Bass. '73.
*Brecher, E. M. and the Editors of Consumer Reports. Licit and illicit drugs. Little. '72.

Brill, Leon and Lieberman, Louis. Authority and addiction. Little.
    '69.
Brown, Wenzell. Monkey on my back. Popular Library. '71.
Burach, Richard. New handbook of prescription drugs. Pantheon.
    '70.
Burke, Evan. Drugs and the turned-on sex generation. Brandon
    House. '73.
Byrd, O. E. Medical readings on drug abuse. Addison-Wesley. '70.
Carey, J. T. The college drug scene. Prentice-Hall. '68.
Carone, P. A. and Krinsky, L. W. Drug abuse in industry.
    C. C. Thomas. '73.
Castaneda, Carlos. The teachings of Don Juan: a Yaqui way of
    knowledge. University of California Press. '68.
Claridge, G. S. Drugs and human behavior. Penguin. '72.
Clark, Janet, pseud. The fantastic lodge: the autobiography of a
    girl drug addict; ed. by H. M. Hughes. Fawcett World Library.
    '71.
    Originally published 1961.
Coles, Robert and others. Drugs and youth. Liveright; Avon. '71.
Collins, Claris and others. Let's talk about drugs: teacher guide-
    lines. Book-Lab, Inc. 1449 37th St. Brooklyn, N.Y. 11218. '73.
Córdova-Rios, Manuel (as told to F. B. Lamb). Wizard of the
    Upper Amazon. Atheneum. '71.
Crowley, Aleister. Diary of a drug fiend. Weiser. '70.
Cuskey, W. R. and others. Drug-trip abroad: American drug-refu-
    gees in Amsterdam and London. University of Pennsylvania
    Press. '72.
Davis, Keith, ed. Drugs and politics. Transaction Books. '74.
Deane, P. G. and Deane, Lola. Is this trip necessary? Nelson-Hall.
    '70.
Deedes, William. The drug epidemic. Barnes & Noble. '71.
Densen-Gerber, Judianne. We mainline dreams: the Odyssey
    House story. Doubleday. '73.
De Ropp, R. S. Drugs and the mind. Grove. '60.
Deschin, C. S. The teenager in a drugged society: a symptom of
    crisis. Richard Rosen Press. '72.
Di Cyan, Erwin and Hessman, Lawrence. Without prescription: a
    guide to the selection and use of medicine you can get over-
    the-counter without prescription, for safe self-medication.
    Simon & Schuster. '72.
Dowling, H. F. Medicines for man: the development, regulation
    and use of prescription drugs. Knopf. '70.
Ebin, David. The drug experience. Grove. '65.
Elgin, Kathleen and Osterritter, J. R. The ups and downs of
    drugs. Knopf. '72.

Emboden, W. A. Jr. Narcotic plants. Macmillan. '72.

Endore, Guy. Synanon. Doubleday. '68.

Falconer, M. W. and others. Current drug handbook. Saunders. '72.

Fiddle, Seymour. Portraits from a shooting gallery: life styles from the drug addict world. Harper. '67.

Fort, Joel. The pleasure seekers: the drug crisis, youth and society. Grove. '70.

*Fremon, S. S. Children and their parents; toward maturity. Harper. '68.

Gallagher, B. G. Campus in crisis. Harper. '74.

Gannon, Frank. Drugs: what they are, how they look, what they do. Warner Paperback Library. '72.

Geller, Allen and Boas, Maxwell. The drug beat. Cowles. '70.

Gimenez, John and Meredith, Char. Up tight! Word Books. '67.

Girdano, D. A. and Girdano, D. D. Drug education: content and methods. Addison-Wesley. '72.

Girdano, D. D. and Girdano, D. A. Drugs: a factual account. Addison-Wesley. '73.

Glatt, M. M. and others. The drug scene in Great Britain; and Journey into loneliness. Williams & Wilkins. '68.

Goode, Erich. The drug phenomenon: social aspects of drug taking. Bobbs. '73.

Gorodetzky, C. W. and Christian, S. T. What you should know about drugs. Harcourt. '70.

Goshen, C. E. Drinks, drugs, and do-gooders. Free Press. '73.

Grinspoon, Lester. Marihuana reconsidered. Harvard University Press. '71.

Hall, Pamela. Heads you lose. Hawthorne Books. '71.

Harms, Ernest. Drugs and youth: the challenge of today. Pergamon. '73.

Hentoff, Nat. A doctor among the addicts. Grove. '70.

Herron, D. M. and Anderson, L. F. Can we survive drugs? 2d ed. Chilton. '72.

Hess, A. G. Chasing the dragon: a report on drug addiction in Hong Kong. Free Press. '65.

Horman, R. E. and Fox, A. M. eds. Drug awareness: key documents on LSD, marijuana and the drug culture. Avon. '70.

Humphreys, Christmas. Concentration and meditation: a manual of mind development. Penguin. '70 .

*Huxley, Aldous. The doors of perception; and, Heaven and hell. (Colophon Books) Harper. '63. 2v in 1.
  Reprinted in this book: Excerpts from The doors of perception (first published in 1954).

Hyde, M. O. ed. Mind drugs. McGraw. '68.

Hyde, M. O. and Hyde, B. G. Know about drugs. McGraw. '71.

Jackson, C. O. Food and drug legislation in the New Deal. Princeton University Press. '70.

Jeffee, Saul. Narcotics: an American plan. Eriksson. '66.

Jones, K. L. and others. Drugs and alcohol. 2d ed. Harper. '73.

Kaplan, E. H. and Wieder, Herbert. Drugs don't take people, people take drugs. Lyle Stuart. '73.

Kaplan, H. I. and Sadock, B. J. eds. Groups and drugs. Dutton. '72.

Kaplan, John. Marijuana—the new prohibition. Harcourt. '70.

Kaplan, Robert. Drug abuse: perspectives on drugs. W. C. Brown. '70.

Kerr, K. A. ed. The politics of moral behavior: prohibition and drug abuse. Addison-Wesley. '73.

Keup, Wolfram, ed. Drug abuse: current concepts and research. C. C. Thomas. '72.

Kiev, Ari. Drug epidemic. Free Press. '74.

Krusich, W. S. and Bradbury, Ralph. Drugs: why unconcerned parents should be concerned. Moody Press. '73.

Land, H. W. What you can do about drugs and your child. Hart. '70.

Larner, Jeremy and Tefferteller, Ralph, eds. Addict in the street. Grove. '65.

Laurie, Peter. Drugs. Penguin. '69.

Leech, Kenneth and Jordan, Brenda. Drugs for young people: their use and misuse. Pergamon. '68.

Leighton, Isabel, ed. The aspirin age: 1919-1941. Simon & Schuster. '63.

Leinwand, Gerald, ed. Drugs. Washington Square Press. '70.

Lessing, Doris. Briefing for a descent into hell. Knopf. '71.

Lieberman, Mark. The dope book: all about drugs. Praeger. '71.

Lindesmith, A. R. The addict and the law. Random House. '65.

Lingeman, R. R. Drugs from A to Z: a dictionary. McGraw. '69.

Linkletter, Art. Drugs at my doorstep. Word Books. '73.

Louria, D. B. The drug scene. McGraw. '68.

Louria, D. B. Nightmare drugs. Pocket Books. '66.

Louria, D. B. Overcoming drugs: a program for action. McGraw. '71.

Lucas, B. G. A B C of drug addiction. Williams & Wilkins. '70.

McCalip, W. C. Jr. and Simon, R. E. Call it fate. Childrens Press. '70.

McCoy, A. W. and others. The politics of heroin in Southeast Asia. Harper. '72.

McGrady, Pat. The persecuted drug: the story of DMSO. Doubleday. '73.

McGrath, J. H. and Scarpitti, F. R. Youth and drugs: perspectives on a social problem. Scott. '70.

Malcolm, A. I. The pursuit of intoxication. Washington Square Press. '72.

Mann, K. W. On pills and needles. Seabury. '69.

Marin, Peter and Cohen, A. Y. Understanding drug use: an adult's guide to drugs and the young. Harper. '71.

Marks, G. J. and Beatty, W. K. The medical garden. Scribner. '73.

Marr, J. S. The good drug and the bad drug. M. Evans. '70.

Matheson, D. W. and Davison, M. A. comps. The behavioral effects of drugs. Holt. '72.

Meyer, R. E. Guide to drug rehabilitation: a public health approach. Beacon Press. '72.

*Mezzrow, Milton ("Mezz") and Wolfe, Bernard. Really the blues. Random House. '46.

Milbauer, Barbara. Drug abuse and addiction: a fact book for parents, teenagers, and young adults. Crown. '70; New American Library. '72.

Moore, Robin. The French Connection: the world's most crucial narcotics investigation. Little. '69.

*Musto, D. F. The American disease: origins of narcotic control. Yale University Press. '73.

Nahal, C. L. ed. Drugs and the other self: an anthology of spiritual transformations. Harper. '71.

Navarra, J. G. Drugs and man. Doubleday. '73.

Nelkin, Dorothy. Methadone maintenance: a technological fix. Braziller. '73.

*Nowlis, H. H. Drugs on the college campus. Doubleday. '69.

Nyswander, Marie. The drug addict as a patient. Grune. '56.

O'Donnell, J. A. and Ball, J. C. eds. Narcotic addiction. Harper. '69.

Olden, Marc. Cocaine. Lancer. '73.

Pace, Denney and Styles, J. C. Handbook of narcotics control. Prentice-Hall. '72.

Palmquist, Al and Reynolds, Frank. Somebody please love me. Bethany Fellowship. '72.

Pekkanen, John. The American connection: profiteering and politicking in the ethical drug industry. Follett. '73.

Pitcaithly, W. L. D. From dope to hope: the story of Father Pit and the Samaritan halfway society, as told to C. Edmund Fisher. Doubleday. '73.

Pope, Harrison, Jr. Voices from the drug culture. Beacon Press. '72.

Proger, Samuel. The medicated society. Macmillan. '68.

Quattrocchi, Frank and Quattrocchi, Henrietta. Why Johnny takes drugs. Aware Press. '72.

Quinn, Barbara. Cookie: the story of an addict. Bartholomew House. '71.

Read, D. A. Drugs and people. Allyn. '72.

Regush, N. M. The drug addiction business: a denunciation of the dehumanizing politics and practices of the so-called experts. Dial. '71.

Rice, Julius. Ups and downs: drugging and duping. Macmillan. '72.

Rosenthal, M. S. and Mothner, I. S. Drugs, parents, and children: the 3-way connection. New American Library. '73.

Russell, Ellen, pseud. Last fix: Dan Russell and the world that lost him. Harcourt. '71.

Saltman, Jules. Drug abuse: what can be done? (Public Affairs Pamphlet no 390A) Public Affairs Committee. 381 Park Ave. S. New York 10016. '72.

Saltman, Jules. The new alcoholics: teenagers. (Public Affairs Pamphlet no 499) Public Affairs Committee. 381 Park Ave. S. New York 10016. '73.

Savary, L. M. ed. Getting high naturally. Association Press. '71.

Scher, J. M. Drug abuse in industry: growing corporate dilemma. C. C. Thomas. '73.

Schmidt, J. E. Narcotics: lingo and lore. C. C. Thomas. '59.

Schoenfeld, Eugene. Dear Doctor Hip Pocrates: advice your family doctor never gave you. Grove. '68.

Seymour, W. N. The young die quietly: the narcotics problem in America. Morrow. '72.

Shedd, C. W. Is your family turned on? coping with the drug culture. Word Books. '71.

Shiller, Alice. Drug abuse and your child. (Public Affairs Pamphlet no 448) Public Affairs Committee. 381 Park Ave. S. New York 10016. '72.

Tully, Andrew. The secret war against dope. Coward. '73.

*Ubell, Earl. The television report: drugs, A to Z. WCBS-TV. 51 W. 52d St. New York 10019. '70.
    Text of series produced by WCBS-TV, New York City.

United States. Marihuana and Drug Abuse Commission. Drug use in America, problem in perspective; 2d report of National Commission on Marihuana and Drug Abuse, March 1973. Supt. of Docs. Washington, D.C. 20402. '73.

WCBS-TV. Drug abuse: what to do . . . where to go if it strikes your child. WCBS-TV. 51 W. 52d St. New York 10019. '72.

Waldorf, Dan. Careers in dope. Prentice-Hall. '73.

Way, W. L. Drug scene: help or hang-up. Prentice-Hall. '70.

*Weil, Andrew. The natural mind: a new way of looking at drugs and the higher consciousness. Houghton. '72.

Weinswig, M. H. Use and misuse of drugs subject to abuse. Bobbs. '73.

Westman, W. C. The drug epidemic: what it means and how to combat it. Dial. '70.

Whitney, E. D. ed. World dialogue on alcohol and drug dependence. Beacon. '70.

Williams, J. B. Narcotics and drug dependence. Glencoe. '74.

Williams, J. B. ed. Narcotics and hallucinogenics: a handbook. Glencoe. '68.

Wise, F. H. Youth and drugs: prevention, detection and cure. Association Press. '71.

Wolfe, Tom. The electric Kool-Aid acid test. Farrar, Straus. '68.

Woodley, Richard. Dealer: portrait of a cocaine merchant. Holt. '71.

Young, W. R. and Hixson, J. R. LSD on campus. Dell. '66.

*Zinberg, N. E. and Robertson, J. A. Drugs and the public. Simon & Schuster. '72.

PERIODICALS

Better Homes and Gardens. 51:18+. Je. '73. Will your child be hooked on drugs? G. M. Knox.

*Chicago Sun-Times. p 10. Jl. 22, '74. Report FBI statistics show 420,000 pot arrests in '73. William Hines.

Chicago Tribune p 11. Ja. 15, '74. U.S. district judge rules army drug control program illegal.

Chicago Tribune. p 14. Ap. 4, '74. Drug information agency, Link, opens in Chicago.

Chicago Tribune. p 2. My. 16, '74. Open Door drug center in Maywood, Ill. described.

Chicago Tribune. p 12. My. 31, '74. Dangers and abuses of prescription drugs. Nicholas Von Hoffman.

Cosmopolitan. 177:96-106. Ag. '74. Girls, doctors and drugs. Arthur Levin.

*Esquire. 39:74-5. Je. '53. How I stopped smoking. Al Hirschfeld.

*Evergreen Review. No 11:15-23. Ja./F. '60. Deposition: testimony concerning a sickness. William Burroughs.

Good Housekeeping. 177:16+. S. '73. Should we turn our son in?

Look. 27:38+. N. 5, '63. The strange case of the Harvard drug scandal. A. T. Weil.

Los Angeles Times. p 13. Ap. 22, '74. Colombia warns travelers of dangers of smuggling drugs.

Los Angeles Times. p 4. Ap. 24, '74. U.S. probes efforts to smuggle Thai marijuana into U.S.

Los Angeles Times. p 2. My. 25, '74. U.S.S.R. issues tough set of
    drug control laws.
Los Angeles Times. p 11. My. 31, '74. N.O. [New Orleans] study
    on aging drug addicts discussed.
McCall's. 100:24. Jl. '73. Rx for families with a drug problem.
Nation. 214:198-9. F. 14, '72. Getting busted abroad. Bernard
    Weiner.
Nation's Business. 62:40. My. '74. Gifts of products help drug ad-
    diction struggle; Phoenix House Foundation. Vernon Lou-
    viere.
New Republic. 165:23-5. Jl. 24, '71. Heroin: the source of supply.
    Eliot Marshall.
*New Republic. 168:13-15. Ap. 21, '73. There's gold in them there
    pills. P. J. Ognibene.
New Times. v 3, no 2:37-40. Jl. 26, '74. Prescription payola.
    Amanda Spake.
New Times. v 3, no 5:35-41. S. 6, '74. Today the seed: tomorrow
    the world. Eleanor Randolph.
New York Post. p 27. Je. 21, '74. Drunkenness losing legal hang-
    over.
*New York Post. p 25. Je. 22, '74. Still problem no. 1. Andrew
    Soltis.
*New York Post. p 1. Jl. 3, '74. Fear surge in heroin supply here.
    Jack Cowley.
*New York Post. p 4. Jl. 5, '74. D.J. takes a dizzy spin so driver's
    won't. W. T. Slattery.
*New York Post. p 10. Ag. 16, '74. Narcotics: another treatment.
New York Post. p 37. Ag. 21, '74. The legal pushers. Carl Rowan.
New York Post. p 3+. S. 4, '74. That tough drug law: the first year.
    Joyce Wadler.
New York Post. p 51. S. 4, '74. A good word for smokers.
New York Times. p 1. F. 19, '72. U.S. report says top drug problem
    is alcohol abuse. H. M. Schmeck, Jr.
New York Times. p 57. Mr. 18, '73. Marijuana found 3rd most
    used drug.
*New York Times. p 1+. Mr. 23, '73. U.S. study stresses treat-
    ment, not penalties. Warren Weaver.
        News analysis: p 19. Drug report: "Liberal law-and-order" view. J. M.
        Markham.
*New York Times. p 58. Mr. 25, '73. Mixing of mind-altering
    drugs rises as spread of heroin addiction slows. J. M. Mark-
    ham.
New York Times. p 31. Ap. 11, '73. Specialists caution legislators
    against isolating the drug problem. F. X. Clines.
New York Times. p 41. Ap. 27, '73. Threat of imprisonment held
    Rx for drug abuse. Lawrence Fellows.

New York Times. p 5. Ja. 15, '74. Court overrules army drug drive.
New York Times. p 30. F. 22, '74. Nixon shifts plan on drug traffic. John Herbers.
New York Times. p 1. Mr. 21, '74. Methadone deaths exceed those from heroin here. M. A. Farber.
New York Times. p 48. Mr. 26, '74. "Victory" over drugs. M. A. Farber.
*New York Times. p 16. My. 5, '74. The poppies of Anatolia [editorial].
New York Times. p 1+. Jl. 11, '74. Alcoholism cost to nations put at $25-billion a year. H. M. Schmeck, Jr.
New York Times. p 1+. Ag. 19, '74. Youths' alcohol abuse called "alarming" here. Enid Nemy.
*New York Times. p 25. Ag. 24, '74. The opium of the people. C. L. Sulzberger.
New York Times. p 9. O. 10, '74. Action by Turkey on poppy lauded; new farm method curbing illicit opium drain-off pleases U.N. officials.
New York Times. p 41+. N. 1, '74. For singles, scene has sordid side. Leslie Maitland.
New York Times. p 1. N. 19, '74. Marijuana found hormone hazard. H. M. Schmeck, Jr.
New York Times. p 24. N. 20, '74. Ford aide backs marijuana curbs. H. M. Schmeck, Jr.
*New York Times. p 47. N. 21, '74. Going to pot. William Safire.
New York Times. p 57. D. 13, '74. Drug use is called on upswing in U.S. Lacey Fosburgh.
New York Times. p 22. D. 28, '74. Harsh penalties for "pot."
New York Times Magazine. p 28-9+. My. 11, '69. A scientific report: the effects of marijuana on human beings. N. E. Zinberg and A. T. Weil.
New York Times Magazine. p 6-9+. Jl. 2, '72. What's all this talk of heroin maintenance? J. M. Markham.
New York Times Magazine. p 108+. N. 19, '72. Overdose explanation is a myth, so why do heroin addicts drop dead? E. M. Brecher.
  Discussion. p 29+. D. 10, '72.
New York Times Magazine. p 56+. Ap. 28, '74. The Wildcat way [supported work program for addicts sponsored by Vera Institute of Justice]. Bruce Porter.
New Yorker. 50:121-4+. N. 18, '74. Smoking still. Thomas Whiteside.
Newsweek. 77:26+. My. 24, '71. GI's other enemy: heroin.
Newsweek. 79:84. Mr. 6, '72. Road to hell. Stewart Alsop.
Progressive. 38:25-9. Ja. '74. Holy war against heroin.

PTA Magazine. 67:20. S. '72. Alternatives to drug use. A. Y. Cohen.

Record (Hackensack, N.J.). p D-1. D. 26, '73. Alcohol re-emerges as nation's biggest drug problem. Sandra Stencel.

*Record (Hackensack, N.J.). p 1. Ja. 28, '74. Pep-pill users: 1 of 3 under 18. Earl Josephson.

Saturday Review. 55:27-32. N. 11, '72. Ups and downs of drug-abuse education. R. H. De Lone.

Saturday Review/World. 1:55-6. Je. 15, '74. Kicking the habit in Japan. Donald Kirk and Susanne Kirk.

Science. 182:40-2. O. 5, '73. The seed: reforming drug abusers with love. Judith Miller.

Science Digest. 74:46. S. '73. Doctors abuse drugs.

Seventeen. 33:146-7+. My. '74. What is Synanon? J. N. Bell.

Society. 10:14-16+. My./Je. '73. The American way of drugging; a symposium.
  Bibliography. p 95.

Sports Illustrated. 36:62-7+. Ja. 24, '72. What made Richie run? Pat Jordan.

Time. 97:18. Je. 21, '71. Heroin shooting war: situation in Detroit.

Time. 101:10. Ja. 15, '73. Lock 'em up; Nelson Rockefeller's proposal of mandatory life sentences for all hard drug pushers.

Time. 102:67+. S. 10, '73. Grass grows more acceptable.

Today's Health. 50:16-19+. Mr. '72. Answers to the most controversial questions about drugs. bibliog D. V. Whipple and Dodi Schultz.

U.S. News & World Report. 73:32. Ag. 7, '72. New progress in the war on drugs.

Vogue. 162:188-9. O. '73. My own devil: the experience of opium smoking. Graham Greene.
  Excerpt from introduction to The quiet American.

Washington Post. Sec C, p 1. Ap. 30, '74. U.S. Supreme Court rules night narcotics searches legal in D.C.

Washington Post. Sec A, p 38. My. 23, '74. Chinese doctor uses acupuncture to treat drug addicts.